Normal Development of Voice in Children

Mette Pedersen

Normal Development of Voice in Children

Advances in Evidence-Based Standards

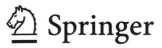
Springer

Dr. Mette Pedersen
Medical Centre
Voice Unit
Ostergade 18-3
1100 Copenhagen
Denmark

ISBN 978-3-540-69358-1   e-ISBN 978-3-540-69359-8

DOI:10.1007/ 978-3-540-69359-8

Library of Congress Control Number: 2008931597

Cover design: eStudio Calamar S.L.

Printed on acid-free paper

9 8 7 6 5 4 3 2 1

springer.com

5/26/09

For my daughter

Preface

The technical measurement of individual parameters in an area as complex as music and song has achieved acceptance only in recent years. However important objective parameters of normal voice development may be, they are especially so when pathological deviations have to be recognised and defined. It is nevertheless also possible to a certain extent to describe different qualities of normal voice development in terms of measurable parameters.

Hormonal changes have a considerable influence on the physical and mental development of boys and girls. The extent to which this influence affects voice development in the two sexes will be made clear in this work through the observation of a number of parameters. I hope that this will stimulate further investigations of this topic. Possible interesting topics for further research are emphasised in the text.

Working with adolescents and documenting their vocal development has given me a lot of pleasure. Colleagues with different medical specialities have supported me in this task. The practical significance of this work has shown itself in the way the results obtained (the graphs and tables) are used today by laryngologists, phoniatricians and music teachers in their daily work, and the determination of hormonal levels in the course of puberty has been introduced as a routine in choirs.

This book is based on a lecture given at the 1991 annual conference of the German Association of Singing Teachers by invitation, and on my thesis, "Biological Development and the Normal Voice in Puberty" (1997). After the presentation in the form of publications in medical journals and as a habilitation thesis, I was encouraged by many people to publish a survey of the results. This was first done in German. In the research project COST 2103 of advanced voice assessment, with 18 countries of the European Union involved, this new updated book records the aspects of voice development in English.

Digitalisation of documents has been performed by Lars Paaske, Copenhagen, and Grit Bühring, Leipzig.

Introduction

The child voice in trained (voice conscious) boys and girls was investigated with phonetograms (voice range profiles) and fundamental frequency (F0) in running speech while reading a standard text. The methods were based on: (1) development and evaluation of the function of phonetograph 8301 made by the firm Voice Profile, and (2) combined electroglottographic and stroboscopic examination of the movements of the vocal folds in speech. The voice analysis was compared with measurements of: (1) pubertal stages in youngsters and (2) hormonal analysis of all androgens and in girls, also estrogens.

The phonetograms (voice range profiles) measured total pitch and loudness range and an area calculation was made of measured semitones x dB(A).

An evaluation was made of the electroglottographic curve, combining it with a marking of the stroboscopic phases of the vocal folds on the curve with a photocell. The electroglottographic single cycles were stable and 2,000 consecutive electroglottographic cycles were measured in 48 boys and 47 girls, aged 8–19 years, to measure fundamental frequency in a reading situation.

Individual and average phonetograms (voice range profiles) for sopranos, altos, tenors and bassos were examined. Careful statistical analysis was made with BMDP on the partly stratified cohort, partly prospective studies.

The yearly change of voice range profiles showed a correlation to total serum testosterone of $r = 0.72$ in the boys, and serum estrone of $r = 0.47$ in the girls.

The change in fundamental frequency in puberty was analyzed in 48 boys. Single observations of the fundamental frequencies showed that total serum testosterone over $10\,nmol\ l^{-1}$ serum represented values for a boy with a pubertal voice.

The voice parameters were analyzed in 47 girls. However, hormonal analysis and pubertal examination were possible only in 41 girls. F0 was related to estrone $r = -0.34$ ($p < 0.05$) only. The increase of estrone and of fundamental frequency range (F0 range) had a predictive value ($p < 0.05$) for the fall of F0 from 256 to 241 Hz in puberty.

The statistical program BMDP was used for all the stratified and prospective studies.

Contents

The Questions to Be Investigated

1

Core Messages

The questions analysed were:

> › How the dynamic range and fundamental frequency change in puberty in boys and girls, in relation to hormonal and all round pubertal biological changes. ■

In collaboration with boys' and girls'choirs and their conductors and vocal instructors, the following questions were devised as the basis for the investigation:

1. How do the tonal range and dynamic range of the voice develop for vocally trained boys and girls?
2. How does the fundamental frequency of the speaking voice develop for vocally trained boys and girls?
3. What is the relationship between the hormonal changes and changes in the trained voice for boys and girls?
4. During which stage of puberty does the trained voice change for boys and girls?

Mette Pedersen, *Normal Development of Voice in Children*
DOI: 10.1007/978-3-540-69359-8, © Springer-Verlag Berlin Heidelberg 2008

Possibilities and Limitations Offered by the Technique Used in the Investigation

2

Core Messages

> The possibilities and limitations of the phonetograms, electroglottograms, electroglottography combined with stroboscopy, fundamental frequency, and register analysis are discussed.

> Phonetograms are called the audiograms of the voice; the dynamic ranges in decibels are compared with their total frequency range.

> Electroglottography is an online quantitative measurement curve of vocal fold closure, based on a high-frequency current of low intensity through the larynx (qualitative also in high speed films with kymography).

> The stroboscopic procedure is supplemented with electroglottography, especially to define the point where the vocal cords close.

> As the closing point is well defined, electroglottography is a good measure for fundamental frequency changes in children and during puberty at the laryngeal level.

Mette Pedersen, *Normal Development of Voice in Children*
DOI: 10.1007/978-3-540-69359-8, © Springer-Verlag Berlin Heidelberg 2008

> › Register changes in pubertal boys were measured
>   with electroglottography and acoustical measurements.
>   The results have been documented with high speed
>   films.

2.1
Phonetogram (Voice Profile) Measurement

Voice profile measurement complements the previously custom-
ary measurement of the tonal range of choir children with a
simultaneous registration of the dynamic range. A standardisation proposal covering this method of investigation from
the Union of European Phoniatricians has been available since
1981 (Seidner and Schutte 1981; Schutte and Seidner 1983). The
form used for documentation of the measurements, which was
developed as part of this proposal and was used in the current
investigation, can be seen in Fig. 2.1.

At the start of our investigations, the measurement of the
dynamic range was performed with a Brüel & Kjær sound intensity meter. The microphone was placed at a distance of 30 cm
from the mouth of the test subject. The test subject first had
to sing the given notes as softly as possible and then as loudly
as possible. The respective sound intensities of the notes were
determined with the sound intensity meter and manually entered
into the documentation forms. However, this type of phonetogram measurement requires some skill, both from the test subject (with respect to exact repetition of the given notes) and from
the investigator (with respect to the instant at which the sound

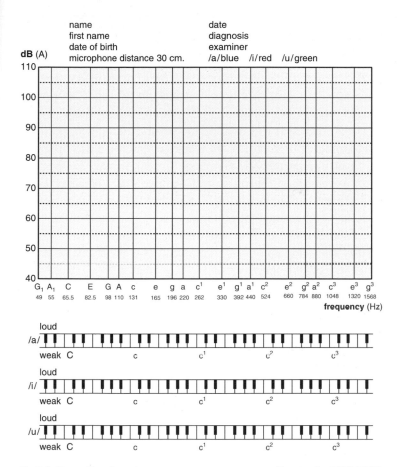

Fig. 2.1 Form for phonetogram measurement according to the 1981 UEP standardisation proposal

2

intensity measurement takes place in the course of the note being sung), and it is also time consuming because of the manual documentation of the results of the investigation.

For these reasons, Pedersen et al. (1984) developed a computer-assisted phonetogram measurement apparatus. The apparatus determines the maximum and minimum intensities of a note as the average over a chosen period of time (0.5–5 seconds), for each semitone, and stores the measured values. The apparatus has been compared with the phonetogram measurement apparatus developed by Wendler and Seidner 1987, Wendler 1989, and the measurements agreed to within 96%. What is new is the exact and defined measurements, and also the standardised caculations of the areas in semitones times decibels and the possibility for averaging of phonetograms in the programs called pg 100 and pg 200 respectively.

The development from the use of conventional to computer-assisted measurements can also be followed in the literature. After a number of publications based on conventional data logging (Bloothooft 1981; Stürzeberger et al. 1982), this apparatus with computer-assisted measurements has increasingly been used (Klingholz and Martin 1983; Seidner et al. 1985; Hacki 1988; Pabon 1991; Kay Elemetrics Corp 1993; Schutte 1995).

The computer-assisted interpretation of the measurement results has also opened up some new possibilities. It is possible to determine the "Average phonetogram" from the phonetogram of several individuals with the pg 200 software, and from this to calculate the standard deviation of the intensity curve (Figs. 2.2 and 2.3; Pedersen et al. 1986a).

The widespread use of phonetograms in phoniatric research is reflected in the literature. Relationships between tone and total intensity (loudness) have been found (Vilkman et al. 1986;

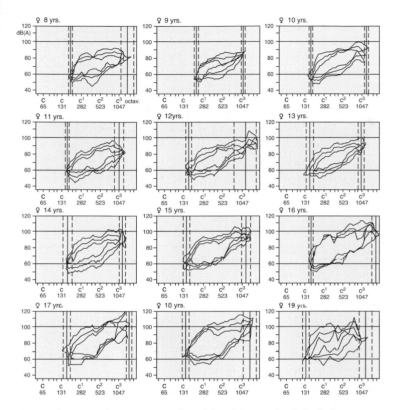

Fig. 2.2 Average phonetograms for girls with standard deviations, as a function of age. The abcissa is divided up into semitones, with the frequency in Hertz for each octave marked. The scale on the ordinate is in dB(A)

Sundberg 1987, 1994). In pathological cases there are intensity variations, which have been discussed by Gramming et al, (1983), Gramming (1988). Hirano (1989) refers to the problem which arises during the investigation of non-musical persons (copying

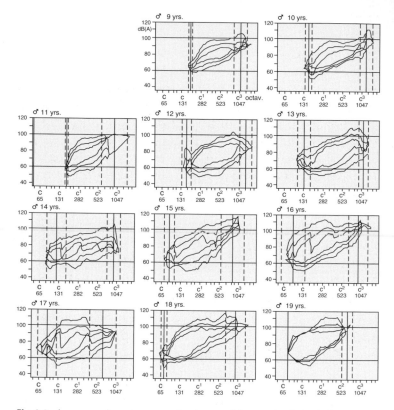

Fig. 2.3 Average phonetograms for boys with standard deviations, as a function of age. The abcissa is divided up into semitones, with the frequency for each octave marked. The scale on the ordinate is in dB(A)

the desired note exactly, holding the note). A technical solution has also been found for this problem, involving making the measurement in half-octave steps and over a shorter time interval or simply measuring the tone given by the patient.

2.2
Electroglottography

Electroglottography was, among others, introduced by Smith (1954) and Fabre (1957) as a procedure for investigating the voice. A high-frequency current of low intensity flows through the larynx between two skin electrodes at the level of the vocal chords. The amplitude modulation of the current due to the changes in resistance during phonation represents the movement of the vocal chords over time. We can follow the use of this method for research purposes over several decades (Loebell 1968; Frokjaer-Jensen and Thorvaldsen 1968; Foucin et al. 1971; Lecluse 1977; Guidet and Chevrie-Muller 1979; Kitzing 1979, 1990, Smith 1981; Hirose et al. 1988; Rothenberg 1992; Hertegård and Gauffin 1995). Dejonckere (1995) gives a review of publications which concern themselves with electroglottography and its uses.

2.2.1
Electroglottography and Stroboscopy

Stroboscopy, which in 1989 – together with other investigative procedures such as phonetogram measurement – was recommended by the International Federation of the Ear–Nose–Throat Associations as a basic method for the diagnosis of diseases of the voice, is not optimal for qualitative investigations of healthy voices. On its own, the stroboscopy method can only be used to distinguish pathological from normal functioning of the vocal chords. However, the method of videostroboscopy is well suited for visualisation of the vibrations of the vocal chords and for displaying the phenomena of the functioning of the larynx, which are generally very difficult to understand (Wendler et al. 1988; Colton et al. 1989, 1995).

As the function of the vocal chords is represented by both electroglottography and stroboscopy, it is worthwhile to use a combination of the two methods to obtain a more complete description of the function of the vocal chords from the parameters, which complement one another. The problem of interpretation of the electroglottography curves (the amplitude and the problem of precisely relating the individual portions of the curve to the phases of the vibration of the vocal chords) can then be solved in a more satisfactory manner. The first results of the combination of stroboscopy and electroglottography were already available when a lively discussion on the interpretation of the glottography curves took place at the International Conference of Logopedics and Phoniatrics in 1974 (Pedersen 1974). Schönhärl had carried out a systematic registration of the stroboscopic data from patients with voice disturbances, but a statistical analysis of the results of treatment was not possible (Schönhärl 1960).

We employed the first simultaneous application of stroboscopy and electroglottography, with an electroglottographic apparatus from the Danish company FJ Electronics in Copenhagen, to investigate music students (trained voices) and hospital workers (untrained voices) (Fig. 2.4; Pedersen 1978). A difference between the two groups could be found in the closing phase of the tone, where the trained voices of the music students showed a larger angular velocity and a shorter duration as it is later shown with kymography. In other respects, the synchronised images of stroboscopy and electroglottography for the two groups were comparable. The electroglottography curve for vocally trained choirboys corresponded to that of the music

Quotients		I 20 hospital employees	II 26 music students
$\dfrac{a}{e}$	av. %	10,5	X 21,2
	s	3,88	3,38
	95% single obs.	2,9-13,1	4,8-37,6
	95% of mean	8,7-13,3	v 17,9-24,5
$\dfrac{a}{b}$	av. %	27,2	X 47,6
	s	12,54	19,41
	95% single obs.	13,7-43,9	9,8-35,8
	95% of mean	21,3-33,1	40,0-63,8
$\dfrac{c}{e}$	av. %	33,8	35,3
	s	7,72	10,81
	95% single obs.	13,7-48,9	6,3-64,3
	95% of mean	30,1-48,9	30,9-39,7
$\dfrac{c}{d}$	av. %	59,6	59,1
	s	13,58	24,33
	95% single obs.	33,0-36,2	10,4-100
	95% of mean	53,2-66,0	49,0-69,1
$\dfrac{b}{e}$	av. %	42,6	44,6
	s	11,93	3,02
	95% single obs.	13,8-65,6	29,1-30,5
	95% of mean	37,2-43,2	41,6-48,0
$\dfrac{f}{e}$	av. %	50,0	X 38,5
	s	10,83	10,34
	95% single obs.	28,8-71,2 diff. P<0.001	19,4-59,8
	95% of mean	44,9-55,1	39,3-42,7

Fig. 2.4 Averages and standard deviations from estimation of electroglottograms, comparing hospital staff (untrained normal voices) and music students (trained voices). The quotients *a/e*, *a/b* and *f/e* are significantly different for the music students, compared to the test persons with untrained voices (cf. Fig. 6)

students in the lower register. Electroglottography is also suitable for the measurement of changes of register. These changes vary depending on the intensity and thus on whether the measurement is carried out from the low to the high register or from high to low (Figs. 2.5–2.7; Pedersen 1977).

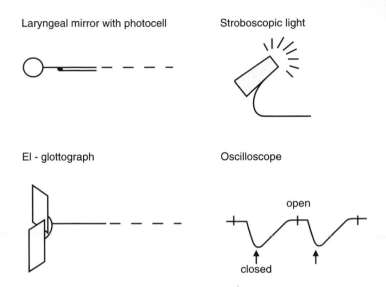

Fig. 2.5 Sketch of the experimental apparatus: Stroboscope, Laryngeal mirror with photocell, Electroglottograph, Oscilloscope

Karnell (1989) and Anastopolo and Karnell (1988) have used our design as the basis for developing an apparatus which makes it possible to combine videostroboscopy and electroglottography. In this way it is possible to compare various individual investigations and to compare average or normal data, to interpret the results of such investigations even more precisely. In addition, clinical use of the method has become possible. This method appears optimal for the representation of the movements of the edges of the vocal chords as described by Smith (1954). Herzel et al. (1994) discuss the non-linear aspects of the movement of the vocal chords. This is further analysed in highspeed films and chaos software, but only in adults. The analysis of differences between

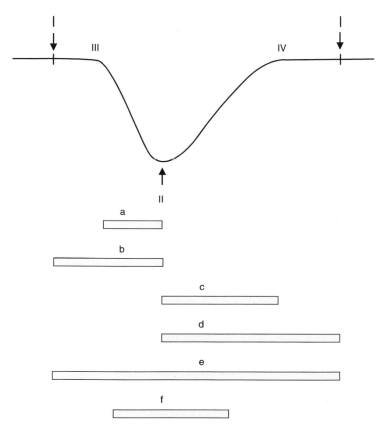

Fig. 2.6 (**I**) Maximum opening of the glottis, (**II**) maximum closing of the glottis (stroboscopically determined and transferred from the electroglottography curve). (**III**) and (**IV**) represent the change in resistance during the transition between these two states (cf. Fig. 4)

the voices of family members has up to now shown no differences which are not frequency dependent, and this has also been demonstrated by muscular studies (Kurita et al. 1980; Kersing 1983).

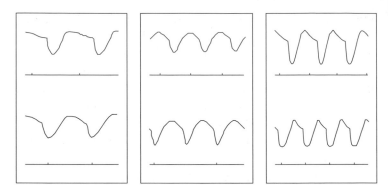

Fig. 2.7 Examples of standard variants of the electroglottography curve. The maximum opening and closing phase were stroboscopically determined and marked on the electroglottography curve

The important function of the maculae flavae was analysed by von Sato and Hirano (1995). In the intervening period, some interesting studies of sex-dependency in the laryngeal musculature appeared (Marin et al 1990; Tobias et al. 1991; Tobias and Kelley 1995; Miranda et al. 1996).

2.2.2
Electroglottography for Determining the Fundamental Frequency of the Speaking Voice

In addition to its use for representing the individual vibrations of the vocal chords, electroglottography is also suitable for the precise registration of the fundamental frequency of the speaking voice Calvet & Malhiac (1950, 1952). We developed a computer program, by means of which this parameter could be calculated from 2,000 electroglottographical cycles. The measurements

took place while a text from the International Phonetic Assoziation (1964), which had been phonetically correctly translated
into Danish ("The North Wind and the Sun"), was being read
aloud. The mean value was given in Hertz. The tonal range of
the speaking voice could be found as the standard deviation in
semitones, so the signals were divided up into semitone windows
from 60 to 684 Hertz (Pedersen et al. 1985a, 1986a, 1990a).

The developed electroglottographic software was presented
in the thesis of Kitzing (1979), and was used for the analysis
of the fundamental frequency of the speaking voice. The company Teltec developed a computerised variant of this apparatus. Roubeau et al. (1987) introduced electroglottography for
the analysis of the fundamental frequency of the speaking voice
for neurological patients. The variation in the fundamental frequency by simultaneous analysis of the histogram configuration
was analysed by Fourchin and Abberton (1971) in phonetics and
Kitzing (1979) in phoniatrics.

Reviews of methods for the measurement of the fundamental
frequency (Baken 1987, Schultz-Coulon and Klingholz 1988)
show that even up to 10–15 years ago the manual estimation
methods of electroglottography were also used for scientific studies. Precise frequency analysis (in combination with jitter and
shimmer), which is made possible by computer assisted evaluation, was performed by von Askenfelt in 1980. The method and
duration of the measurements were discussed by von Karnell
(1991). In the age of computer assisted speech perception (Pahn
and Pahn 1991), precise measurements should no longer be a
problem (Elman and Zipser 1988; Rihkanen et al. 1994). With
the use of neural networks, the possibility of determining the
relationship between the fundamental frequency and blood flow
in the brain arises (Sataloff 1995; Pedersen 1991b, 1995). From

these investigations, it will perhaps be possible to achieve a better understanding of the central control of voice.

2.3
Tone and Register Analysis

A Brüel & Kjær sound analyser and a Nicolet Ubiquitous 44A spectral analyser were used for the analysis of formant production. This analysis was presented at the International Conference of Logopedics and Phoniatrics in 1977, and demonstrated that the 12 13 year old test subjects in a boys' choir had a high singing formant of on average 5,000 Hz.

Auditive investigations were traditionally used for recording the changes between registers. In our investigations these tasks were dealt with by the music teacher.

A video film with stroboscopy of Danish choirboys, during puberty, performed with the von Timcke stroboscopy apparatus from Medizinische Hochschule in Hannover, was presented at the Voice Symposium held in Manhattan School of Music, New York, (Pedersen et al. 1988). This illustrates the difficulties of capturing the changes in the vibrations of the vocal chords during puberty. Stroboscopy is more suitable for qualitative documentation of register changes than phonetograms or electroglottography (Svec and Pesak 1994; Vilkman et al. 1995). Both the last-named methods have been employed for the quantitative recording of changes of register (Seidner and Wendler 1982; Frokjaer-Jensen 1983).

Although the objective of this work was not primarily tonal analysis of trained pubertal voices, the documentation of formant analysis in childhood nevertheless appears interesting (Sundberg

1987). Formant production during puberty is subject to several influences, such as for example the conditions for the investigation, physical and hormonal development and vocal technique. Still, focussing on the harmonics gives more secure statistical results, especially in pathology.

For boys, the changes of register during puberty, like the fundamental frequency of the speaking voice and the lowest tone of the tonal range, depend on the testosterone level. For girls, no analysis of this phenomenon has been available up to now. The relationships between hormonal changes and development of the voice during puberty for girls have been investigated for the first time by our research group.

Materials and Method

3

Core Messages

› 48 boys and 47 girls were systematically analysed in a stratified study at a choir school. A basic test of capability of reproducing tones and rhythms was made at the entrance to the choir.

› Phonetograms were made with the standardization of the Union of European Phoniatricians.

› Fundamental frequency was based on 2,000 cycles of electroglottographical measurements.

› Hormone measures included serumtesterostone, dehydroepiandrosteron, delta-4, androsteron, oestradiol, oestrone, and oestrone sulphate plus sex hormone binding globulin. The five pubertal stages were measured.

› The BMDP statistical programme based on logarithms was used for the one-way multivariate analysis and prospective aspects.

Mette Pedersen, *Normal Development of Voice in Children* 19
DOI: 10.1007/978-3-540-69359-8, © Springer-Verlag Berlin Heidelberg 2008

3

3.1
Test Persons

48 boys and 47 girls took part in the transverse study. 4–5 pupils
came from each form, with their ages ranging from 8 to19 years.
All of them were put through a musicality test, which included
reproducing a rhythm by clapping (Wöldike's test), repeating
notes by singing, and singing a given song with high notes
(Fig. 3.1a and b). All these tests were of a type well known to
the pupils, used for determining the type of voice. Stroboscopic

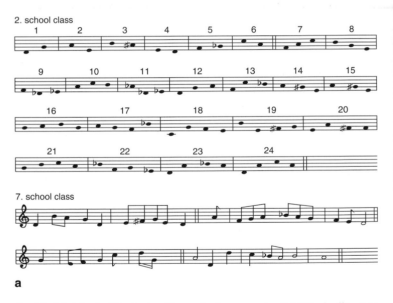

a

Fig. 3.1 (**a**) Musicality test – Reproducing a note. (**b**) Musicality test
– Wöldike's rhythm test

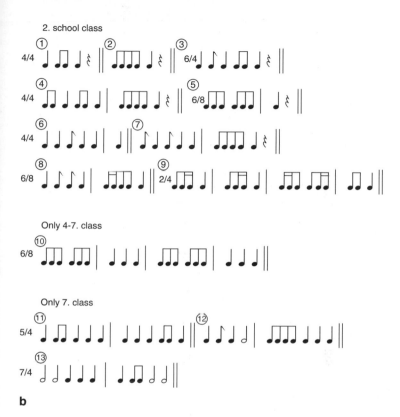

Fig. 3.1 (continued)

analysis showed normal data for all of them. The stage of puberty was judged by a paediatrician to be typical for the age of each pupil (Pedersen 1991c; Brook 1995).

3.2
Method of Investigation

3.2.1
Phonetogram Measurement

Measurement of phonetograms was performed in accordance with the standardisation proposal from the Union of European Phoniatricians, 1981. The lowest note, the middle note and the phonetogram areas in semitones × dB(A) [ST × db(A)] were recorded for statistical evaluation. Before we had the possibility of computer supported phonetogram evaluation, we performed the calculation of the phonetogram areas by means of planimetry (lcm^2 = 32 ST × dB(A)). The tonal range was given in semitones, to maintain a logarithmic scale on both the abscissa and the ordinate, to avoid errors in the statistics. A normal school room was used for the investigation. All the data were stored in the computerised phonetogram apparatus (with a transportable IBM PC), (Pedersen et al. 1984, 1986b).

3.2.2
Measurement of the Fundamental Frequency

The fundamental frequency of the speaking voice was registered by electroglottography and averaged over 2,000 cycles by using a computer. From the mean value of the frequency in Hertz, the fundamental frequency was worked out; the tonal range during the flow of speech was also averaged to give the tonal range of the speaking voice. As specified in Section 2.2.2 the measurement took place as a given text was being read out. A model 830 electroglottograph from the company FJ Electronics, a model

2208 noise meter, a model 5066 Brüel & Kjær stroboscope and a Tectronix oscilloscope were used.

3.2.3
Hormonal Status and Pubertal Analysis

The hormonal analysis was based on those parameters which to our knowledge change earliest in the course of puberty. Children from the age of 8 were included in the investigation, as the adrenarche (increased prepubertal function of the adrenal glands at this age) will possibly provide information which will help us to understand puberty. The following values were analysed: Serum testosterone (free and total, there is a close relationship between the two values), dihydroepiandrosterone (DHEAS), delta-4-androsterone and the transport globulin for testosterone, the Sex-Hormone-Binding-Globulin (SHBG). For the girls, the program of investigation also included the following parameters: Oestradiol (E2), oestrone (E1) and oestrone sulphate (E1SO4). The build-up and working period of androgens and oestrogens are complex, and the same is true of the possible interactions between the individual hormones. After we had attained some insight into the relationships between hormonal changes and voice development by means of these investigations, we would have liked to have included all the androgen regulating hormones in the hypothalamus in the investigation, so as to have more precise results. It is to be hoped that our work can provide the starting point for more detailed hormonal brain research in the future.

In addition, body size and weight, testicle volume, the stage of pubic hair development and (for girls) the stage of breast development were determined for each of the test subjects (Pedersen et al. 1985a; Brook 1995).

3.2.4
Statistical Analysis

Measurement results do not have any scientific value before they have been subjected to statistical analysis to determine their significance. The first problem was the question of whether linear or logarithmic relationships should be used. The logarithmic criteria that were used, based on geometric cross sections, are considerably stricter than the linear ones. A one-way multivariate analysis was performed, using the fundamental frequency of the speaking voice as classifier to determine whether there were differences between the groups. For all variables we determined the correlation coefficients, to be able to calculate the relationships between them and their dependency on age by using the partial correlation coefficients. The BMDP statistical program was used.

Results

4

Core Messages

> Phonetograms (planimetry) had clearly bigger dynamics in the older pupils after the pubertal register shift, with a falling of the lowest tones in both sexes.

> The fundamental frequency in reading a standing text changed in boys with an octave and in girls with one-fourth octave, related significantly to an increase of the tonal range of five semitones for both girls and boys.

> The statistically significant results are that the change of fundamental frequency in puberty is related to testosterone in boys and estrogens in girls.

> Prospectively testosterone values over 10 nmol/ml suggest a boy in vocal puberty. A girl after menarche and with a tonal range in reading of five semitones is postpubertal.

Mette Pedersen, *Normal Development of Voice in Children*
DOI: 10.1007/978-3-540-69359-8, © Springer-Verlag Berlin Heidelberg 2008

4.1
The Phonetogram in the Course of Voice Development

Figure 4.1 shows the development of the phonetograms during puberty for boys (Pedersen et al. 1986). In puberty, the area of the phonetogram is smaller and the changes of register are

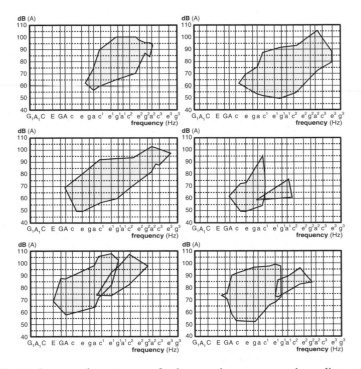

Fig. 4.1 Average phonetograms for boys and young men, depending on voice type. (The voice type was determined by the singing teacher.) The range of the artistically usable singing voice is marked on the abcissa. (A: Beginner, B–C: Soprano, D: Alto, E: Voice in puberty, F–G: Tenor, H–I: Bass)

altered. After puberty, the lowest note lies deeper, and the areas of both the lower and the upper registers increase.

The phonetograms of girls likewise show changes during puberty (Fig. 4.2). At the beginning of puberty they demonstrate modest changes, but then at the age of about 14.5 years, as in the case of boys, alterations in the change of registers take place (Pedersen et al. 1990).

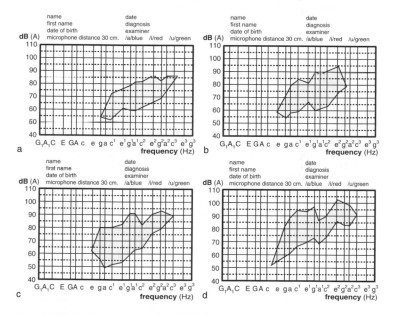

Fig. 4.2 Phonetograms for girls of different ages. (**a**) (8.9 years) – Beginner in the choir. (**b**) (11.7 years) – Typical child's voice with change of register (330–392 Hz). (**c**) (13.8 years) – Well-trained voice without register changes with limited dynamic breadth. (**d**) (14.8 years) – Pubertal voice with register changes

For the transverse study, we divided the male subjects into 3 groups: pre-pubertal, pubertal and post-pubertal voices. The phonetograms of the groups differed significantly ($p < 0.01$) with respect to the areas, the lowest note and the tonal range. The same is true for the fundamental frequency, for serum testosterone and for SHBG (Fig. 4.3, Pedersen et al. 1986).

For female subjects, there were significant differences between the 3 groups (pre-pubertal, pubertal and postpubertal) with respect to the phonetogram areas, the lowest note and the tonal range of the speaking voice. For the average fundamental frequency of the speaking voice, however, no significant differences between the groups could be seen. For oestrogen and oestrone sulphate, we found significant differences ($p < 0.001$); this was also the case for androstendione and DHEAS, but not for SHBG (Fig. 4.4, Pedersen et al. 1990).

The phonetogram areas for boys changed depending on the volume of the testicles, corresponding to the serum testosterone level. The changes in the phonetogram areas during puberty are however a very complex matter, where age-related development also plays a decisive role (Fig. 4.5, Pedersen et al. 1986).

The development of girls' voices shows noticeable differences compared to boys. For girls, the average fundamental frequency of the speaking voice changes independently of the phonetogram areas ($r = 0.29$), whereas for boys the dependency between these two parameters persists ($r = 0.50$). For the tonal range of the speaking voice, there are no differences between the two sexes, both are related (girls: $r = 0.54$; boys: $r = 0.49$). The changes in the phonetogram areas depend on the stage of pubic hair development for girls ($r = 0.51$) and for boys ($r = 0.65$). For girls there is also a connection to breast development.

Voice category	Voice category group	Number of boys	Age of years	Phonetogram area cm²	Fo/Fo range Hz/semitones	Tone range semitones	SHBG nmol/1	Pubic hair stage	Free testosterone nmol/1
Non-differentiated beginners	I	5	9.1	13.0	287/3.6	30.3	112	1.0 (1)	0.0019
1. Soprano	II	5	11.3	20.6	254/4.3	37.7	123	1.6 (1-2)	0.0254
2. Soprano	III	7	12.0	25.5	266/4.2	35.8	132	2.1 (1-4)	0.0194
Alto	IV	10	12.3	25.2	259/3.4	33.9	130	2.1 (1-4)	0.0210
Puberty	V	4	14.9	23.3	144/5.0	35.2	56	4.3 (3-5)	0.21
1. Tenor	VI	2	18.0	29.2	141/4.7	40.5	46	5.0 (5)	0.42
2. Tenor	VII	6	16.8	34.7	131/5.2	41.1	33	5.2 (3-5)	0.47
1. Bass	VIII	7	17.5	35.2	127/4.8	42.7	42	5.4 (5-6)	0.26
2. Bass	IX	2	16.5	30.0	109/6.2	39.1	48	5.3 (5-5.3)	0.32
Mutual SD within groups (f = 39) in percent of mean				37	7	17	61		315

Fig. 4.3 Comparison between male voice types in the transverse study with respect to phonetogram area, fundamental frequency of the speaking voice, tonal range of the singing voice in semitones, SHBG, stage of pubic hair development and free testosterone, in boys

Group	1	2	3	5	6	7	SD significancy
Age	11.1	11.6	12.7	15.9	16.4	17.8	
Number	3	11	5	5	6	3	
Weight (KG)	36	40	56	59	60	65	
Mamma stage	1	1-3	2-4	3-5	4-5	4-5	
Phonetogram area (cm^2)	16.2	18.0	22.4	24.2	26.1	33.2	432 < 0.01
Fundamental frequency in ct. sp. (Hz)	248	261	229	249	253	229	11 NS
Tone range in ct. speech (semitones)	3.74	4.31	3.77	5.41	4.70	4.58	21 < 0.01
Tone range in singing (semitones)	33.0	34.2	33.7	35.1	35.7	40.9	10 NS
Phonetogram (Hz)							
Lowest tone	185	162	145	167	148	136	12 NS
Middle tone	466	432	365	465	391	431	14 < 0.05
Highest tone	1245	1165	1022	1288	1163	1449	22 NS
E1 (p-mol)	65.6	59.4	75.7	151.5	126.2	126.4	46 < 0.001
E1S04 (p-mol)	703	901	1214	2378	2438	2618	115 < 0.001
E2 (p-mol)	71.6	79.6	95.1	170.4	101.9	94.0	115 NS
Androsten dione (n-mol)	1.22	1.94	1.75	3.94	3.21	3.61	138 < 0.05
DHEAS (n-mol)	4200	3500	2900	4700	5900	7600	68 < 0.01
Total-testosterone (n-mol)	0.79	0.67	0.46	0.92	0.98	0.70	86 NS

Fig. 4.4 Geometrical averages of vocal and hormonal parameters for different voice types in the female group (8–19 years). 1: Child's voice 1st. Soprano, 2: Child's voice 2nd. Soprano, 3: Child's voice Alto, (4: Mutating voice (no values shown)), 5: Adult voice 1st. Soprano, 6: Adult voice 2nd. Soprano, 7: Adult voice Alto. SD – Standard deviation of the average value. Significance calculated using t-test. Groups 1–3 versus groups 5–7.

Voice parameters	Age	Phonetogram area
Total tone range	0.48	0.63
Fo in fluent speech	−0.86	−0.50
Voice range	0.58	0.54
Lowest frequency	−0.87	−0.62
Middle frequency	−0.73	−0.34
Puberty		
Axillery hair stage	0.84	0.58
Pubic hair stage	0.89	0.65
Testis volume	0.87	0.71
Height	0.90	0.64
Weight	0.86	0.60
Hormones		
Total testosterone	65.6	0.72
Free testosterone	703	0.69
Dihydrotestosterone	71.6	0.69
Delta-4-androstendione	1.22	0.76
DHEAS	4200	0.59
SHBG	0.79	- 0.41

r 00.6 age/phonetogram area
All p < 0.01 except middle frequency/phonetogram area

Fig. 4.5 Logarithmic correlation coefficient for different vocal and hormonal parameters in relation to age and phonetogram area, respectively

Increase in body weight is recognised as a normal phenomenon in puberty. The correlation between the development of the phonetogram areas and somatic changes during puberty is significant for both sexes in the case of the stage of pubic hair development, of body weight and for girls also of breast development. With respect to the hormonal parameters, androgens play a significant role, both for girls and for boys. For girls, a significant correlation could also be found between oestrone and oestrone sulphate and the development of the phonetogram areas. For the body size of girls, there is no significant age dependency, while all other parameters change in proportion to age (Fig. 4.6 and 4.7. Pedersen et al. 1990a and b).

Figure 4.8 gives a graphical representation of how the changes in voice category for boys are related to the falling level of SHBG and the rising level of serum testosterone. There are also correlations between testicle volume, the stage of pubic hair development and the phonetogram areas (Pedersen et al. 1986a and b).

Similar phenomena are seen for girls. Here the voice changes are related to androstendione, oestrone, body weight and the stage of pubic hair development (Fig. 4.9, Pedersen et al. 1990a and b).

For boys, the average annual changes were evaluated, for example, the fundamental frequency of the speaking voice (11%) and the phonetogram areas (9.2%) (Fig. 4.10). Another interesting parameter is the deepest note of the phonetogram, which falls to a similar extent to the fundamental frequency of the speaking voice (12%). The androgen level rises to an extent comparable to which the level of SHBG falls (Pedersen et al. 1982).

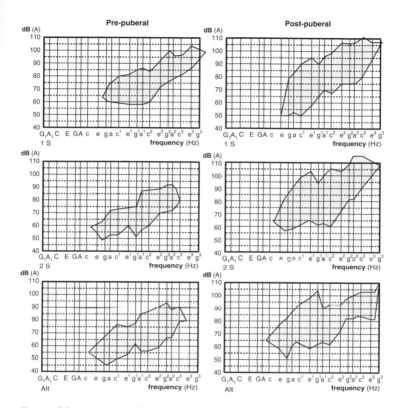

Fig. 4.6 Phonetograms for girls of different voice types. In the upper frequency range, there is a bigger intensity for the sopranos, and in the lower frequency range for the altos.

Voice	Age	Phonetogram area
Total tone range in singing	0.44 **	0.66 **
Fundamental frequency in continuous speech	−0.44 **	−0.29 **
Tone range in continous speech	0.59 ***	0.49 ***
Lowest frequency	−0.57 ***	−0.58 ***
Middle frequency	−0.30 **	−0.15 **
Puberty		
Axillery hair stage	0.61 ***	0.41 ***
Pubic hair stage	0.76 **	0.51 **
Mamma development stage	0.48 ***	0.38 ***
Menarch, time after	0.52 ***	0.29 ***
Weight	0.69 **	0.48 **
Height	0.22 ***	0.20 ***
Hormones		
Total testosterone	0.49 ***	0.32 ***
Delta-4-androstendione	0.57 ***	0.39 ***
DHEAS	0.66 ***	0.38 ***
Oestrone (E1)	0.74 ***	0.47 ***
Oestradiol (E2)	0.35 *	0.20 *
Oestrone sulphate (E1SO4)	0.69 ***	0.44 ***

Significance: $p < 0.05$ ($r >$ or $= 0.30$): *
                  $p < 0.01$ ($r >$ or $= 0.39$): **
                  $p < 0.001$ ($r >$ or $= 0.49$): ***

Fig. 4.7 Correlation coefficients of different vocal and hormonal parameters in relation to age and phonetogram area for girls (age/phonetogram area: $r = 0.65$)

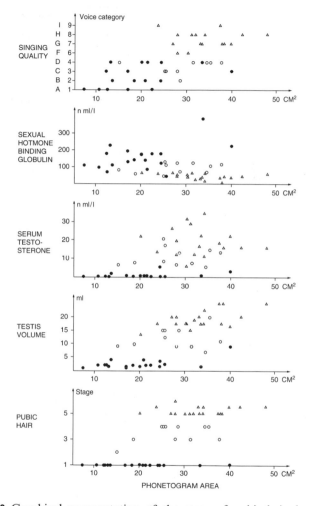

Fig. 4.8 Graphical representation of the stage of pubic hair development, testicle volume, serum testosterone level (total), SHBG and voice type (A – I, see Fig. 4.9) for boys as a function of phonetogram area (abcissa): (*filled circle*) 8.7–12.9 years, (*open circle*) 13–15.9 years, (*open triangle*) 16–19.5 years. (1 cm^2 = 32 semitones x dB(A))

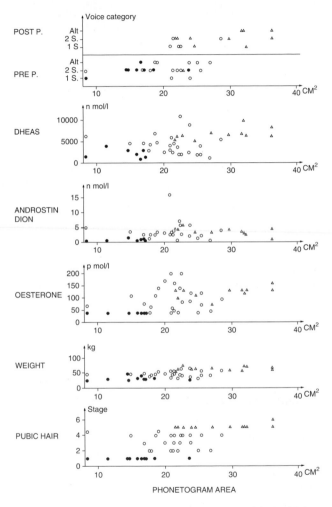

Fig. 4.9 Graphical representation of the parameter with the highest correlation with phonetogram area (1 cm² = 32 semitones x dB(A)) for girls: (*filled circle*) Breast development stage 1, (*open circle*) Breast development stage 2–4, (*open triangle*) Breast development stage 5–6

Age	(years)	8.7-12.9	13.0-15.9	16.0-19.5	pr yr. % change
No of boys		19	15	14	
Serum testosterone	(n mol/l)	0.54	10.5	18.9	68
Dihydrotestosterone	(n mol/l)	0.18	1.21	1.57	37
Free testosterone	(n mol/l)	0.007	0.14	0.33	77
Sexual hormone binding globulin	(n mol/l)	134	66	45	−16
Delta 4 androstene dione	(n mol/l)	0.54	1.17	2.5	24
Dehydro epi andro sterone sulfate	(n mol/l)	1400	4100	5900	25
Testist volume	(ml)	2.3	13	20	36
Fundamental frequency	(Hz)	237	184	125	−11
Voice range	(semitones)	3.7	4.8	5.0	3.9
Phonetogram area	(cm^2)	19	28	34	9.2
Lowest biological tone	(Hz)	158	104	72	−12

Fig. 4.10 Geometrical average of hormonal, pubertal and vocal parameters for boys (grouped according to age) and the annual change in these parameters in %. (Phonetogram area: 1 cm^2 = 32 semitones x dB(A))

4.2
The Speaking Voice in the Course of Voice Development

The fundamental frequency of the speaking voice is by itself a frequently investigated parameter used for describing the development of the voice. This fact explains the previous assumption that girls' voices hardly change during puberty. As mentioned in Section 4.1 above, there is for girls no significant correlation between the fundamental frequency of the speaking voice and the phonetogram areas; however, there are correlations between the phonetogram areas, the deepest note of the phonetogram and the tonal range of the speaking voice. For boys, the fundamental frequency gets deeper with age in a manner parallel to that of the deepest note of the phonetogram and at the same point in time as the tonal range of the speaking voice and the phonetogram areas rise, while at an age of about 14.5 years a reduction in the phonetogram areas takes place (Fig. 4.11, Pedersen et al. 1986a and b).

The change in the fundamental frequency of the speaking voice for girls is – given in Hertz – smaller and less pronounced than the change in the deepest note in the phonetogram. For girls, too, there is an increase in the phonetogram areas (for the post-pubertal group of girls $28.3 \, cm^2 = 895.6 \, ST \times dB(A)$: for the post-pubertal group of boys $34 \, cm^2 = 1088 \, ST \times dB(A)$, with the conversion factor $1 \, cm^2 = 32 \, ST \times dB(A)$). The clearest changes take place in the tonal range of the speaking voice (post-pubertal group of girls 5 ST, boys 5.2 ST), as shown in Fig. 4.12 (Pedersen et al. 1990a and b, 1986a and b).

A commonly overlooked fact is that the physiological changes have significantly larger physical effects for girls. The fundamental frequency of the speaking voice for girls changes from 256 Hz in the pre-pubertal group to 241 Hz in the post-pubertal group. The tonal range of the speaking voice increases from its pre-pubertal value of 3.7 ST to a post-pubertal value of 5.2 ST; these changes are significant to 99%. In parallel with this, the serum oestrone level (E1) rises from 57 to 123 pmol/l (pico means nano/1000).

Body weight was on average for the youngest group of girls 37.8 kg and for the oldest group 64.4 kg. In the age group of 8.6–12.9 year old girls, 4 out of 18 had already reached menarche; in the age group of 16–19.5 year olds, all the girls had (Fig. 4.13, Pedersen et al. 1990a and b). There was a linear correlation

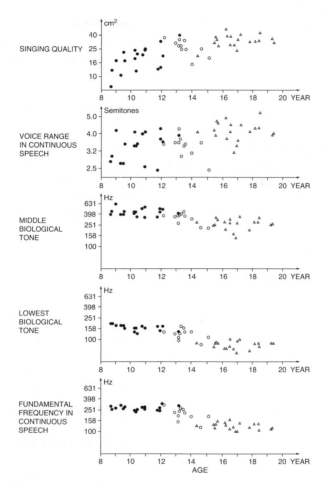

Fig. 4.11 Graphical representation of the phonetogram areas, the tonal range of the speaking voice, the deepest and the mean note in the phonetogram and the fundamental frequency of the speaking voice for boys as a function of age (abcissa): (*filled circle*) 8.7–12.9 Jahre, (*open circle*) 13–15.9 Jahre, (*open triangle*) 16–19.5 Jahre

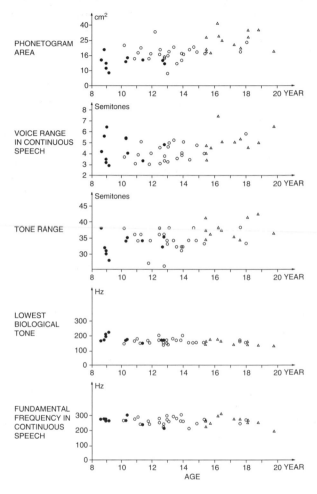

Fig. 4.12 Graphical representation of vocal parameters (phonetogram areas, tonal range of the speaking voice, tonal range of the singing voice, deepest note in the phonetogram, fundamental frequency of the speaking voice) for girls as a function of age (abcissa): (*filled circle*) Breast development stage 1, (*open circle*) Breast development stage 2–4, (*open triangle*) Breast development stage 5–6

Age	(years)	8.7-12.9	13.0-15.9	16.0-19.8	Significance
Total number		18	12	11	
Oesterone (E1)	pmol	57	104	123	**
Oestradiol (E2)	pmol	73	135	108	
Total testosterone	nmol	0.5	0.76	0.94	
Free testosterone	nmol	0.006	0.037	0.009	
Oesterone sulphate (E1SO4)	pmol	732	1924	2342	**
DHEAS	nmol	3210	3700	7200	**
Androstendione	nmol	1.44	3.28	3.43	*
Sex hormone binding globulin (SHBG)	nmol	153	130	123	
Menarche		+4	+9	+11	
Pubic hair stage		1-4	2-5	4-6	
Mamma development stage		1-4	2-5	5	
Fundamental frequency in continuous speech	Hz	256	248	241	
Tone range in continuous speech	Semitones	3.7	4.2	5.2	**
Tone range in singing	Semitones	23	30	38	
Phonetographic area	cm^{2*}	17.3	21.8	28.3	**
Phonetogram lowest tone	Hz	166	156	145	*
Phonetogram middle tone	Hz	429	409	413	
Phonetogram highest tone	Hz	1136	1105	1263	

* cm^2 conversion factor: 1 cm^2 = 32 semitones*dB(a).

Fig. 4.13 Geometrical averages of hormonal, pubertal and vocal parameters for girls (grouped by age). The relative standard deviation lay between 11% and 140%. (Significance of the differences between the groups: $p < 0.01$ xx; $p < 0.05$ x)

between the SHBG level and the arrival of menarche for girls ($r = 0.93$); this correlation could however not be confirmed if the statistical calculation was based on logarithmically transformed values (Pedersen et al. 1987).

4

Figure 4.14 shows the fundamental frequency of the speaking voice for boys compared to the stage of pubic hair development, to testicle volume, to serum testosterone and to SHBG (Pedersen et al. 1986a and b). In an earlier pilot study (Pedersen et al. 1982) of 25 boys, we were able to demonstrate that the fundamental frequency of the speaking voice is high until the age of 13, and that for the age group of 13–15 year olds the fundamental frequency is also still above 195 Hz, while the serum testosterone level has already risen to up to 10 nmol l^{-1}. Not until we reach the age group of 15 years does the fundamental frequency of the speaking voice fall to below 150 Hz, while the serum testosterone level of this age group is at least 10 nmol l^{-1}. The high serum testosterone level shows a correlation either with the falling tonal range in the high notes or to more distinct changes of register. All young men of 17–18 years had an adult tone of voice. The average fundamental frequency of the speaking voice lay 8–12 semitones above the deepest note in the phonetogram (Fig. 4.15).

The changes of register for boys lay – as determined auditively by music tearchers with practised ears – around 627 Hz in group 1 (age 11.8–13.2 years; testosterone < 1 nmol l^{-1}) and around 649 Hz in group 2 (age 13.2–14.7 years; testosterone < 10 nmol l^{-1}). In the group of 14.8–16.9 year olds, the change of register had fallen with a significance of 99% to an average of 312 Hz (standard deviation 70 Hz) (Pedersen and Munk 1983) (Fig. 4.16).

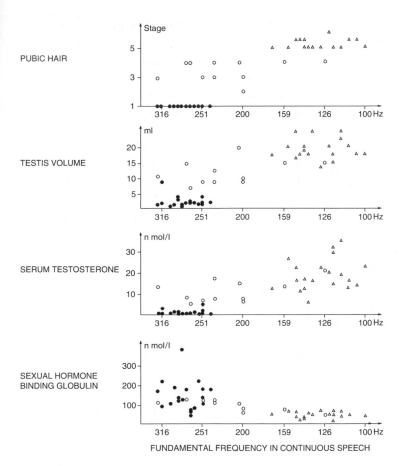

Fig. 4.14 Graphical representation of the stages of pubic hair development, testicle volume, serum testosterone (total) ande SHBG for boys as a function of the fundamental frequency of the speaking voice (abcissa): (*filled circle*) 8.7–12.9 years, (*open circle*) 13–15.9 years, (*open triangle*) 16–19.5 years

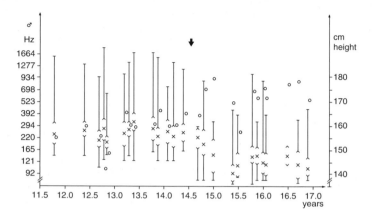

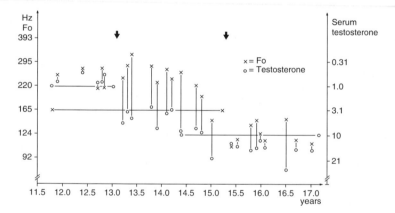

Fig. 4.15 Above: Fundamental frequency of the speaking voice, tonal range of the speaking voice and tonal range of the singing voice for boys compared to body height (ordinate) and age (abcissa). *Below:* Fundamental frequency of the speaking voice [Hz] compared to serum testosterone level [nmol l⁻¹]. The abcissa shows the age in years. The arrows indicate the change of voice (*above*: End of the change; below: Beginning and end of the change)

TONERANGE	Bioloical tonerange			Lower (reg)	Higher for singing
♂	χ/SD	χ/SD	χ/SD	χ/SD	χ/SD
Group I	136.4	1302.0	190.40	627.67	990.50
< 1 nmol Serumtestosterone	(20.5)	(690.06)	(22.46)	(216.5)	(208.5)
Group II	124.17	1223.30	174.78	649.86	990.0
< 10 nmol Serumtestosterone	(31.0)	(893.01)	(44.22)	(154.7)	(276.2)
Group III	79.74	471.22	86.02	321.56	723.57
> 10 nmol Serumtestosterone	(5.4)	(287.44)	(12.97)	(70.4)	(366.12)

Fig. 4.16 Changes of register for boys, grouped according to serum testosterone level (I <1 nmol l^{-1}; II <I0 nmol l^{-1}; III >I0 nmol l^{-1}). The tonal range of the singing voice is given here first as the biological range and second as the artistically usable tonal range; the difference between the two was calculated (reg means average register change)

4.3
Further Results from the Statistical Analysis

Good statistical methods appear also to be useful in music and song research for drawing strong conclusions from the results of analysis.

With our material, we have – with respect to the average fundamental frequency of the speaking voice – performed a one-way multivariate analysis, and this has enabled us to predict the timing of the change of voice in relation to the hormonal and bodily changes in the individual case (Fig. 4.17, Pedersen et al. 1985a and b). For boys in the group at stage 2–4 of pubic hair development and an average age of 13.5 years, a correlation between the lowering of the average fundamental frequency of

Number of boys	Stage of puberty	Geometrical mean values			Coefficient	
		x̄ Fo Hz	age	λ̄ SHGB nmol	age	log SHGB
18	1	274	10.5	141	0.0002	0.010
11	2-4	219	13.5	91	− 0.0016	0.501*
19	5-6	129	16.9	42	− 0.0014	0.005
48	Total				− 0.0033	0.171*

Fig. 4.17 Predictive coefficient of boys, the fundamental frequency of the speaking voice and age, hormonal parameters and stage of puberty, evaluated within the framework of a multiple regression analysis. Independent parameters are not included. Mean value of the remaining parameters according to grouping. *Coefficient is significantly different from zero ($p < 0.05$)

the speaking voice and the falling SHBG level was found. This means that a drop in the fundamental frequency can be expected when the SHBG level falls in those pubescent stages. For girls, there was a significant correlation between a falling fundamental frequency and an increasing level of serum oestrone ($p < 0.05$) and oestrone sulphate, as well as the tonal range of the speaking voice ($p < 0.05$), independent of age. Before menarche, there exists a correlation between the fundamental frequency and the level of oestrone sulphate, body size and the stage of development of pubic hair. After menarche, a highly significant dependency ($p < 0.001$) appeared of the tonal range of the speaking voice and also of the period of time which had passed since menarche. The larger the tonal range of the speaking voice, the lower the fundamental frequency for the speaking voice of girls in puberty (Figs. 4.18 and 4.19, Pedersen et al. 1990a and b).

	Fo	/Fo tone range	Lowest tone	Age
Oesterone (E1)	−0.34 *	/0.40 **	−0.35 *	0.74 **
Oestradiol (E2)	−0.21	/0.10	−0.18	0.35 *
Total testosterone	−0.08	/0.36 *	−0.34 *	0.49 **
Free testosterone	−0.17	/0.27	−0.40 **	0.52 **
Oesterone sulphate (E1SO4)	−0.18	/0.32 *	−0.29	0,69 **
DHEAS	−0.17	/0.40 **	−0.24	0,66 **
Androstendione	−0.19	/0.30	−0.35	0,57 **
Sex hormone binding globulin (SHBG)	0.06	/0.05	−0.14	0.30
Menarche time after beginning	−0.06	/0.33 *	−0.14	0.52 **
Pubic hair stage	−0.19	/0.53 **	−0.46 **	0.76 **
Mamma development stage	−0.08	/0.37 *	−0.34 *	0,48 **
Height	0.06	/0.26	−0.15	0.22
Weight	−0.22	/0.51 **	−0.44 **	0.69 **
Fo in continuous speech	−	−	−0.51 **	−0.40 **
Tone range in continuous speech	−0.07	−	−0.28	0,59 **
Tone range in singing	0.10	/0.45 **	−0.46 **	0.44 **
Phonetographic area	−0.29	/0.49 **	−0.58 **	0.65 **
Phonetogram lowest tone	0.51 **	/−28	−	−0.57 **
Phonetogram middle tone	0.45 **	/0.05	0.71 **	−0.30
Phonetogram highest tone	0.14	/0.33 *	0.08 **	0,08

The correlations to the lowest tone in the phonetogram and age are also shown (significance: ** P < 0.01, * P < 0.05).

Fig. 4.18 Correlation coefficients, between the fundamental frequency of the speaking voice and the tonal range of the speaking voice for girls, compared to the female sex hormones, androgens, stage of pubic hair development, stage of breast development and vocal parameters. The table also shows the correlation between the deepest note of the phonetogram and age (Significance: $p < 0.01$ xx; $p < 0.05$ x)

All girls		Pre - menarche		Post - menarche	
Variable	P- value of t-test	Variable	P- value of t-test	Variable	P- value of t-test
Weight	0.066	Height	0.001 ***	Age	0.033 *
Log (tone range in speech)	0.042 *	Pubic hair (stage)	0.022 *	Time after menarche	0.008 **
Log (E1)	0.054	Log (E1SO4)	0.001 ***	Log (tone range in speech)	0.001 ***
Log (E1SO4)	0.043 *			Log (androst)	0.068
S.E. of estimation	0.034	0.0166	0.0288		
S.D. of log	0.037	0.0300	0.0409		
F-test: P- value	0.0443	0.0006	0.0036		

Linear correlation coefficient SHBG, r - 0.93 to menarche. * P < 0.05; ** P < 0.01; *** P < 0.001.

Fig. 4.19 Predictive correlation of the fundamental requency of the speaking voice for girls, evaluated for all test persons and divided into two groups (before and after menarche). Linear correlation coefficient of **SHBG** with Menarche $r = 0.93$ Significance: $p < 0.05$ x $p < 0.01$ xx $p < 0.001$ xxx

Discussion

5

Core Messages

> Knowledge of the hormonal aspects of voice is necessary in highly qualified choirs and in pathology as well.

> Phonetograms may make pupils conscious about their qualifications and can be measured before and after treatment of pathological cases.

> Phonetograms can be "beautiful", showing smooth variations for low and high intensities with no register shift, e.g. sopranos in the Thomaner choir in Leipzig.

> The fundamental frequency development is an interesting biological parameter in puberty and the basis for mathematical models, e.g. in technology, biology, brain research and telecommunications.

Mette Pedersen, *Normal Development of Voice in Children*   **49**
DOI: 10.1007/978-3-540-69359-8, © Springer-Verlag Berlin Heidelberg 2008

5.1
Hormonal Status and Pubertal Analysis

Puberty is defined as the period of time during which the ability to reproduce is attained. In practice, it is related to the development of the secondary sexual characteristics. The normal development of humans during puberty is a very complex process. Brook (1995) has produced a survey article which is partly based on an investigation by Tanner and Whitehouse (1976). For Brook (1995), the development of the voice is described as "the breaking of the voice" at the age of about 14.5 years, and the definite attainment of an adult voice about a year later. Potassium metabolism increases in close relationship to the level of sexual hormones, and also depends more on the stage of puberty than on age (Krabbe 1989). The body size of Danish children was reported on by Andersen (1968) and later by Roed et al. (1989) and Hertel et al. (1995), and matches our measurements.

Brook (1995) maintains that knowledge of the development of the heart and lungs is limited, and the development of these organ systems until now has only been related to body size and to the development of the secondary sexual characteristics. Similar remarks apply to the paediatric literature on voice development. Hägg and Taranger (1982) characterise the voice as childish, pubertal or adult, Karlberg and Taranger (1976) describe the breaking of the voice in relation to the stage of puberty at an age of 14.5 years, and Heinemann's work is concerned with abnormal processes in the development of the voice during puberty (1976). Kahane (1982) analyses the development of the thyroid cartilage in relation to body size, and Hirano et al. (1983, 1988) have measured the growth of the vocal chords during the time of puberty.

Normal endocrinological development is controlled by the gonadotropin-releasing hormone from the hypothalamus (Brook 1995). Through the influence of this decapeptide, LH and FSH are released from the frontal lobes of the hypophysis. They regulate the growth of the testes and the ovaries. The sexual hormones are produced by these organs. Our methods of measurement have been described by Lykkesfeldt et al. (1985). The measurements are comparable to those of other authors (Apter and Vihko 1985). A review of the function of SHBG has been given by Strel'Chyonok and Vihko (1985), among others.

With the method by means of which one can perform hormonal analysis on saliva, possibilities are open for investigating the close relationship between hormonal changes and voice (Walker et al. 1993). New insights into the relationships between cerebral regulation and the development of the voice in physiological and pathological cases (Young et al. 1988; Walker et al. 1993) will also make it possible in the future to explore the phenomenon of the change of voice from a neurophysiological point of view (Rodriguez-Sierra 1986; Behre and Nieschlag 1995; Nastiuk and Clayton 1995). One further perspective of this is that we may expect to discover new aspects of our understanding of the psychology of music (Seashore 1938; Pedersen 1992; Dejonckere et al. 1995). Niedzielska et al. (1999) compared change of voice with pathological activation of the gonades in male puberty. Abitbol et al. (1999) found that the harmonics are hormonally dependent in male and female puberty. Breteque and Sanchez (2000) analysed the deepening of the speaking voice in boys and showed the individual nature of the related change of the singing voice. Charpy (2002) underlines the concept that voice breaking does exist in adolescent females. Chernobelsky (2002) shows that electroglottograms are highly effective in training vocal registers in deaf children also.

Wiskirska-Wonica et al (2006) studied delay of voice break in adolescent boys. Van Lierde et al. (2006) found no statistical significant difference for females, using the dysphonia severity index (DSI) between resonance parameters in the menstrual cycle in 24 healthy young profesional voice users.

5

5.2
The Phonetogram in the Course of Voice Development

The development of the voice during puberty was also investigated in the current work within the framework of a stratified (transverse) cohort study. Longitudinal prospective studies have in this context the advantage that intra-individual comparisons are also performed. For this reason we have investigated 3 boys over the period of one year (from the end of the 7th school grade to the end of the 8th grade). Measurements were carried out every two months. The six phonetograms for one of the boys are shown in Fig. 5.1 (Pedersen 1993). The average phonetograms for the three boys before and during the change of voice were also worked out with our phonetography software (pg200, means and SD) (Fig. 5.2). The start of the change of voice happened for all 3 boys during their 8th school year. The vocal changes during this year were not dependent on age. The deepest note in the phonetogram, which our previous investigations had shown to be highly correlated with the fundamental frequency of the speaking voice, was significantly dependent on the SHBG level. Thus SHBG showed itself also in this study to be the most sensitive parameter for the lowering of the frequency of the voice. As only the limited segment of the entire period of puberty was

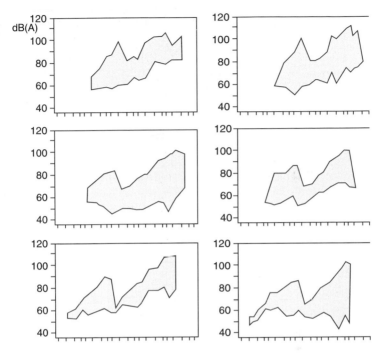

Fig. 5.1 6 phonetograms, measured on a boy at intervals of two months (age 13.7–14.6 years). The third phonetogram (December) has the biggest area and shows the smallest irregularities. In January, the boy was suspended from singing in the choir due to the start of the change of voice ($C4 = 262$ Hz)

investigated, no significant relationships between the changes in the phonetogram areas and testosterone level were found. With respect to the serum testosterone level, there is during this stage of puberty considerably more inter-individual variation than in earlier or later stages. The phonetogram areas likewise change

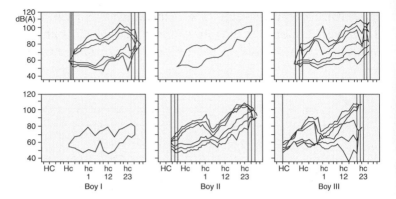

Fig. 5.2 Average phonetograms and standard deviations for the three choirboys (I–III) involved in the prospective longitudinal study. The phonetograms before and after the change of voice were compared. For test person I and II, only one phonetogram was made in mutation and before mutation respectivetly. For test person III, three phonetograms were measured before and three during the change of voice

markedly over a short period of time: the phonetogram simply becomes more irregular and the changes of register appear more distinctly. Attempts to give a mathematical description of the irregularities (by a characteristic number for the phonetogram, or a fractal dimension) have, however, so far not produced any satisfactory results; incorporation of these values in the statistical calculations was not meaningful (Bühring and Pedersen 1992, Arainer and Klingholz 1993).

To assess the possible influences of local peculiarities on the Copenhagen subjects, either on the vocal parameters or on hormonal values, we performed an investigation of some members of the Leipzig Thomanerchor (Group 1: boy sopranos, before the change of voice; Group 2: those whose voices had just broken), where 4 subjects were investigated in each group (Fig. 5.3). Looking at the phonetograms of the Copenhagen boys and girls, we see an enlargement of the phonetogram

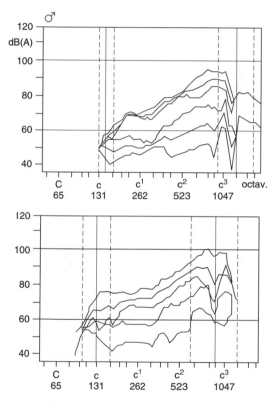

Fig. 5.3 Average phonetograms with standard deviation for the cohort of sopranos and of pubertal change groups (mutants) from the Leipzig Thomaner choir. The hormonal parameters were similar to those of the Copenhagen boys

areas for group 1 (pre-pubertal) compared to group 3 (post-pubertal). During puberty (at an age of 14.5 years), the areas of the phonetograms became temporarily smaller (Figs. 5.4 and 5.5). The soprano group of the Thomaner choir was comparable to the soprano group of the Copenhagen boys with respect to the deepest note and the phonetogram areas, whereas the highest note of the Thomaner sopranos lay higher than that of the Copenhagen sopranos. These differences are possibly due to a stricter selection of choir members or a better technical mastery of the voice. In the average phonetograms of both Thomaner groups, there is also a very small standard deviation in the forte curve, larger in the range of the changes of register.

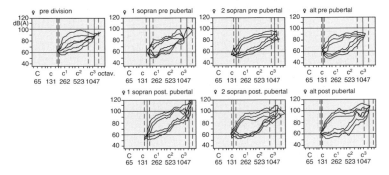

Fig. 5.4 Average phonetograms with standard deviation for girls and young women from a girls' choir at a Danish choir school, as a function of voice type. (The voice type was determined by the singing teacher.) The abcissa is divided up into semitones, and the frequency in Hertz of each octave is indicated. The scale of the ordinate is dB(A). One group could not be securely defined during puberty

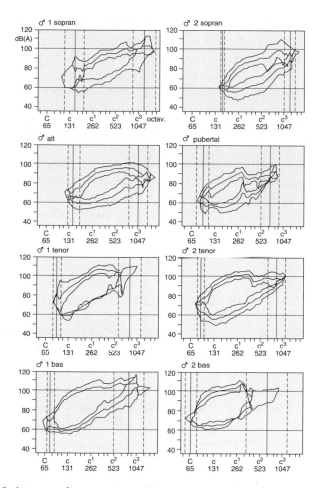

Fig. 5.5 Average phonetograms with standard deviation for boys and young men from a boys' choir at a Danish choir school, as a function of voice type. (The voice type was determined by the singing teacher.) The abcissa is divided up into semitones, and the frequency in Hertz of each octave is indicated. The scale of the ordinate is dB(A)

We also performed a pilot study of the Thomaner boys on electroglottographical determination of the changes of register. The boys first sang a rising chromatic scale as softly as possible and then as loudly as possible; during this process, the electroglottogram was drawn. With respect to hormonal values, there was no difference between the Leipzig and the Copenhagen subjects (Behrendt and Pedersen 1989; Pedersen 1991c).

Before the use of phonetograms as a method for simultaneous registration of the tonal and dynamic range of voice, the development of the voice was only described by the tonal range. Already at an early stage in the history of phoniatrics, investigations of the tonal range for normal school children were carried out (Flatau and Gutzmann 1905). A summary of the results of research into children's voices was proposed at the Conference of Logopedics and Phoniatrics in 1936, and subsequently performed by Weiss (1950). This summary covers a period of 4,000 years and shows that people concerned themselves almost exclusively with boys' and eunuchs' voices. The average age for the change of voice was 14.5 years; the fundamental frequency of the speaking voice for boys dropped by about an octave and for girls by about 1/3 octave. Frank and Sparber (1970) and Wendler and Seidner (1987) arrived at comparable results. Blatt (1983) discusses the topic of voice training during puberty.

Komyama et al. (1984) performed an analysis of phonetograms during puberty. They did not, however, make any comparisons with other pubertal phenomena, and fixed the lower measurement limit for intensity at 60 dB. In our investigations, the intensity of the voice during soft singing was significantly lower, and thus the measurements are not comparable.

Meuser and Nieschlag (1977) showed that the type of voice for men (tenor, baritone, bass) is related to the serum testosterone level. Large and Iwata (1972) found differences between the formants which depended on the voice type for adults. We also believe that a distinction between the types of voice must be made, if an exact appraisal of the development of the voice during the time of puberty is to be achieved. This could in the future possibly also be considered in investigations of the pathology of the voice. Pedersen et al. (1980) made a follow up on voice disorders.

During the period of our investigations, Klingholz et al. (1989) carried out phonetograms on members of the Tölzer boys' choir; in addition, Konzelmann et al. (1989) investigated the phonetograms of choirboys. A summary of the literature can be found in the work of Bühring (1990). Behrendt (1989) followed the development of the falsetto register of the boys of the Thomaner choir until the age of adulthood, but did not relate the phenomena to other parameters.

Hacki (1988, 1989) used the shouting voice measurements in phonetograms. Phonetograms help in the work of music teachers and performers. With this method, it is possible to check the results of instruction on the regulation of dynamics (especially during soft singing) and the changes of register more precisely, also in choirs (Bonet and Casan 1994; McAllister et al. 1994; Böhme and Stuchlik 1995; Sulter et al. 1995). The voice however cannot be assessed independently of other bodily functions (Pedersen 1991a, Krusnevskaja and Pedersen 1992) (Fig. 5.6).

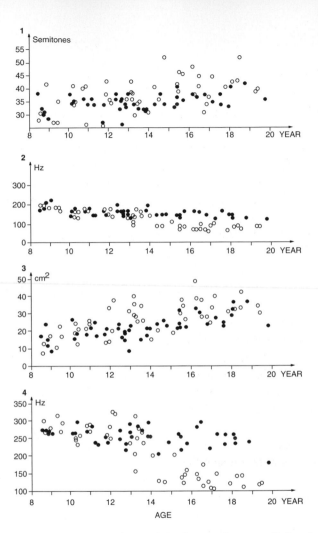

Fig. 5.6 Age related comparison of 1. the tonal range of the singing voice, 2. the deepest note, 3. and the area of the phonetogram, 4. and the fundamental frequency of the speaking voice for the two sexes: (*filled circle*) girls, (*open circle*) boys (1 cm² in the area = 32 Semitones x dB(A))

5.3
The Speaking Voice in the Course of Voice Development

Summaries of the scientific work which relates to the fundamental frequency of the speaking voice in children have been made by Baken 1987 and Schultz – Coulon et al. 1988. Among others, Fairbanks et al. 1949, Michel et al. 1966, Hollien and Malcik 1967; Hollien and Shipp 1972; Hollien 1983; Hollien et al. 1994; Fitch and Holbrook 1970; McGlone and McGlone 1972 and Coleman et al. 1977 have studied the development of the fundamental frequency of the speaking voice in children, without however also investigating the tonal range of the speaking voice. Vuorenkoski et al. (1978) have compared the average fundamental frequency of the speaking voice with hormonal levels in children with endocrinological diseases. Bastian and Unger (1980) investigated the fundamental frequency of the speaking voice in the different stages of puberty. Harries et al (1998) used laryngographic measurements on boys and found a good correlation between the sudden drop in frequency seen between Tanner stages 3 and 4. Lundy et al. (2000) used the singing power ratio as an objective means of quantifying the singers' formant; the values were not significantly different between the sung and spoken samples in young singing students. In the literature there are not, however, many studies in which the process of bodily maturation in connection with hormonal development has been related to the important secondary sexual characteristic which the voice constitutes. Barlow and Howard (2002, 2005) used the closed quotient with electrolaryngographic measurements on 127 children with measurable effect on training. Amir et al. (2002) and Amir and Biron-Shental (2004) showed that it is a good idea to make supplemental sex hormone evaluation in different medical vocal conditions. They also showed that oral contraceptives might stabilise the voice. Cheyne et al (1999) suggest normative values for electroglottography.

The voice is naturally not only an interesting biological parameter in puberty, but also during the menopause. Truuverk and Pedersen (1992) investigated the phonetogram of the speaking voice and its relationship to androgen and oestrogen in amateur female choir singers in the World Festival Choir. A connection was found between high oestradiol and a larger area in the phonetogram for the speaking voice. Russell et al. (1995) analysed the tonal range of the speaking voice in adult women and obtained similar results. Chan (1994) documented by electroglottography improvements in the voices of trained kindergarten teachers.

It is possible that calculations based on new mathematical models (Titze 1994, Siegel 1994) can reveal unknown aspects of hormonal regulation of the voice (Blaustein 1986, Miranda et al. 1996). This would also be interesting for the quantitative differentiation between physiological and pathological voice development (Andersson-Wallgren and Albertsson-Wikland 1994; Byrne, Dillon & Tran (1994); Yukizane et al. 1994). For voice research, the employment of technologies and the interpretation of the measurement results from a biological point of view are of the greatest importance.

Answers to the Questions Posed

6

Core Messages

> Phonetrograms increase in both sexes, except for a temporary decrease of dynamics and range between 13.5 and 14.5 years of age. The specific voice changes in both sexes depend on the sex hormonal level. Sex hormone binding globulin falls, predicting the drop of one octave of the fundamental frequency in boys. After menarche the expansion of the tonal range and the increasing level of estrogen sulphate predict the fundamental frequency change in girls. For both sexes the change of voice is measured maximally between 13.5 and 14.5 years of age.

Phonetograms and electroglottography provide important measurements which – when interpreted in conjunction with other parameters – can expand our understanding of the way in which the development of the voice proceeds.

In the light of the information which we have accumulated from our investigations, we can answer the questions which we posed at the start of this work in the following way:

Mette Pedersen, *Normal Development of Voice in Children*   63
DOI: 10.1007/978-3-540-69359-8, © Springer-Verlag Berlin Heidelberg 2008

1. How do the tonal and the dynamic ranges of the voice develop for vocally trained boys and girls?

   The phonetogram areas in simitones times db(A) increase gradually for both sexes in the course of puberty. However, they temporarily decrease in the age range between 13.5 and 14.5 years; this phenomenon is more pronounced for boys than for girls.

2. How does the fundamental frequency of the speaking voice develop for vocally trained boys and girls?

   The speaking voice changes in both sexes during puberty. For boys, the change is dependent on the serum testosterone level, and for girls on the oestrone level. In the male group, the average fundamental frequency of the speaking voice drops, while in the group of girls the tonal range of the speaking voice expands.

3. What are the relationships between hormonal changes and changes in the trained voice for boys and girls?

   The voice changes during puberty, depending on the testosterone level and the oestrone level respectively for boys and girls, and independently of age. The falling level of SHBG precedes the drop in the fundamental frequency of the speaking voice in boys. These changes take place during stages 2–4 of puberty, and also during this period the testosterone level rises. For girls, the drop in the fundamental frequency of the speaking voice follows the increasing levels of oestrone and oestrone sulphate and the expanded tonal range of the speaking voice.

4. During which stage of puberty do the trained voices of boys and girls change?

   The timing of puberty and the way in which it proceeds are different for boys and girls; nevertheless, the changes in the voice take place for both sexes between 13.5 and 14.5 years. Until now it has not been possible to set up famous girls' choirs in the same way as boys' choirs. Apart from reasons of tradition, limited knowledge of girls' voices and the way in which they change during puberty has played a role in this. To achieve an optimal development of musical expression for girls, one should take into consideration that the speaking voice must lie in the biologically determined frequency range that is correct for each individual, and not too high (Collin and Koppe 1995).

References

Abitbol, J., Abitbol, P., Abitbol, B. (1999) Sex hormones and the female voice. J. voice 13(3): 424–446

Airainer, R. & Klingholz, F. (1993) Quantitative evaluation of phonetograms in the case of functional dysphonia. J. Voice 7: 136–141

Amir, O. & Biron-Shental, T. (2004) The impact of hormonal fluctuations on female vocal folds. Curr. Opin. Otolaryngol. Head Neck Surg. 12(3): 180–184

Amir, O., Kishon-Rabin, L., Munchnik, C. (2002) The effect of oral contraceptives on voice: preliminary observations. J. Voice 16(2): 267–273

Amy de la Breteque, B. & Sanchez, S. (2000) A comparative acoustic study of the speaking and singing voice during the adolescent's break of the voice. Rev. Laryngol. Otol. Rhinol. (Bord) 121(5): 325–328

Anastopolo, S. & Karnell, M.P. (1988) Synchronized videostroboscopy and electroglottography. J. Acoust. Soc. Am. 83: 1883–1890

Andersen, E. (1968) Skeletal maturation of danish school children in relation to height, sexual development and social conditions. Acta Paediatr. Scand. Suppl. 185: 64–72, 98–101

Andersson-Wallgren, G. & Albertsson-Wikland, K. (1994) Change in speaking fundamental frequency in hormone-treated patients with Turner's syndrome – a longitudinal study of four cases. Acta Paediatr. Scand. 83: 452–455

Apter, D. & Vihko, R. (1985) Premenarcheal endocrine changes in relation to age at menarche. Clin. Endocrinol. 22: 753–760

Askenfelt, A., Gauffin, J., Sundberg, J. & Kitzing, P. (1980) A comparison of contact microphone and electroglottography for the measurement of vocal fundamental frequency. J. Speech Hear. Res. 23: 258–273

Baken, R.S. (1987) Clinical Measurement of Speech and Voice. College Hill, Boston, pp 197–240

Barlow, C. & Howard, D.M. (2002) Voice source changes of a child and adolescent subjects undergoing singing training – a preliminary study. Logoped Phoniatr. Vocol. 27(2): 66–73

Barlow, C. & Howard, D.M. (2005) Electrolaryngographically derived voice source changes of children and adolescent singers. Logoped Phoniatr. Vocol. 30(3–4): 147–157

Bastian, H.-J. & Unger, E. (1980) Untersuchungen des Zusammenhangs von Akzeleration, Mutation und Dysphonie anhand von Längsschnittuntersuchungen. Arztl. Jugendkd. 71: 205–211

Behre, H.M. & Nieschlag, E. (1995) Biological effects of testosterone: new aspects. Eur. J. Clin. Invest. 25(Suppl. 2): A 49

Behrendt, W. (1989) Auditive Beurteilung des Stimmklanges mànnlicher Fistelstimmen bei ehemaligen Chorknaben. Sprache, Stimme, Gehor 13: 60–63

Behrendt, W. & Pedersen, M. (1989) A comparative pubertal study of Thomaner choir, Leipzig and Copenhagen boys choir. Oral presentation at Voice Symposium, Philadelphia

Blatt, J.M. (1983) Training singing children during the phase of voice mutation. Ann. Otol. Rhinol. Laryngol. 92: 462–468

Blaustein, J.D. (1986) Steroid receptors and hormone action in the brain. Ann. N. Y. Acad. Sci. 474: 400–413

Bloothooft, G. (1981) Voice profiles, vowel spectra and vocal registers. Proc. IXth Congress Union of European Phoniatricians. Amsterdam. 1981: 83–85

Bohme, G. & Stuchlik, G. (1995) Voice Profiles and Standard Voice Profile of Untrained Children. J. Voice 9: 304–307

Bonet, M. & Casan, P. (1994) Evaluation of dysphonia in a childrens choir. Folia. Phoniatr. 46: 27–34

Bretéque, A.B. & Sanchez, S. (2000) A comparative acoustic study of the speaking and singing voice during the adolescent's break of the voice. Rev. Laryngol. Otol. Rhinol. (Bord) 121(5): 325–328

Brook, C.G.D. (ed.) (1995) Clinical Endocrinology. 3rd edn, Blackwell, Oxford

Bühring, G. (1990) Die Anwendung der CAD-System: CADy bei der Computergestützten Stimmfeldwertung. Dissertation A. Leipzig

Bühring, G. & Pedersen, M.F. (1992) Fractal dimensions of phonetograms, a stratified and longitudinal study during development of male voices. Proc. XXIlnd Congr. Int. Ass. Logoped. Phoniatr. 1: 1–9

Byrne, D., Dillon, H. & Tran, K. (1994) An international comparison of long-term average speech spectra. J. Acoust. Soc. Am. 96: 2108–2120

Calvet, J. & Malhiac, G. (1952) Courbe vocales et mue de la voix. Congres Bull. Soc. Fr. Foniatr. (1950) and J. Fr. Otorhinolar. 1: 115–124

Chan, R.W.K. (1994) Does the voice improve with vocal hygiene education? A study of some instrumental voice measures in a group of kindergarten teachers. J. Voice 8: 279–291

Charpy, N. (2002) Voice breaking phenomenon in female adolescents. Rev. Laryngol. Otol. Rhinol. (Bord) 123(5): 297–301

Chernobelsky, S. (2002) The use of electroglottography in the treatment of deaf adolescents with puberphonia. Logoped. Phoniatr. Vocol. 27(2): 63–65

Cheyne, H. A. Nuss, R.C. Hillman, R.E. (1999) Electroglottography in the pediatric population. Arch Otolaryngol Head Neck Surg. 1999; 125:1105–1108.

Coleman, R.F., Mabis, J.H. & Hinson, J.K. (1977) Fundamental frequency – sound pressure level profiles of adult male and female voices. J. Speech Hear. Res. 20: 197–204

Collin, F. & Koppe, S. (ed.) (1995) Humanistisk Videnskabsteori (Humanistic science theory). Danish Radio, Copenhagen

Colton, R.H., Casper, J.K., Brewer, D.W. & Aronson, D.G. (1989) Digital processing of laryngeal images: a preliminary report. J. Voice 3: 132–142

Colton, R.H., Woo, P., Brewer, D.W., Griffin, B. & Casper, J. (1995) Stroboscopic signs associated with benign lesions of the vocal folds. J. Voice 9: 312–325

Dejonckere, P.H. (1995) Electroglottography: a useful test in voice evaluation. 1st. World Conf. of Voice, Portugal. Abstract book: 136

Dejonckere, P.H., Hirano, M. & Sundberg, J. (1995) Vibrato. Singular publishing group, San Diego

Elman, J.L. & Zipser, D. (1988) Learning the hidden structure of speech. J. Acoust. Soc. Am. 83: 1615–1626

Fabre, P. (1957) Un precode electrique percutane d'inscription de l'accolement glottique au cours de la phonation glottographie de haute frequance. Premiers resultats. Bull. Acad. Natl. Med. 121: 66

Fairbanks, G., Wiley, J.M. & Larsman, F.H. (1949) An acoustical study of vocal pitch in seven and eight-year-old boys. Child. Dev 20: 63–69

Fitch, J.L. & Holbrook, A. (1970) Modal vocal fundamental frequency of young adults. Arch. Otolaryngol. 92: 379–382

Flatau, T.S. & Gutzmann, H. (1905) Die Singstimme des Schulkindes. Arch. Laryngologie 20: 327–348

Fourchin, A.J. & Abberton, E. (1971) First application of a new laryngograph. Med. Biol. Illus. 21: 172–182

Frank, F. & Sparber, M. (1970) Stimmumfang bei Kindern aus neuer Sicht. Folia Phoniatr. 22: 397–402

Frokjaer-Jensen, B. (1983) Can electroglottography be used in the clinical practice. Proc. XIXth Congr. of IALP, Edinburgh. vol II: 849–851

Frokjaer-Jensen, B. & Thorvaldsen, P. (1968) Construction of a Fabre Glottograph. ARIPUC. Copenhagen University, Denmark 3: 1–8

Gramming, P. (1988) The phonetogram. Thesis. University of Lund, Sweden

Gramming, P., Pedersen, M. & Kitzing, P. (1983) Datoriserade fonetogram for objectivering av rost funktions storninger. Lakar stamman/Stockholm. Otolaryngologisk section (oral presentation)

Guidet, C. & Chevrie-Muller, C. (1979) Computer analysis of prosodic and electroglottographic parameters in diagnosis of pathologic voice. In: Winkler, P. (ed.) Investigations of the speech process. Quantitative linguistics. Dr. Brockmeyer Studienverlag, Bochum. 19: 233–261

Hacki, T. (1988) Die Beurteilung der quantitativen Sprechstimmleistungen. Das Sprechstimmfeld. Folia Phoniatr. 40: 190–196

Hacki, T. (1989) Klassifizierung von Glottisdysfunktionen mit Hilfe der Elektroglottographie. Folia Phoniatr. 41: 43–48

Hägg, U. & Taranger, T. (1982) Maturation indication and the pubertal growth spurt. Am. J. Orthod. October: 299–309

Harries, M., Hawkins, S., Hacking, J., Huges, I. (1998) Changes in the male voice at puberty: vocal fold length and its relationship to the fundamental frequency of the voice. J Laryngol Otol. 112(5): 451–454

Heinemann, M. (1976) Hormone und Stimme. J. Ambrosius Barth Verlag. Leipzig.

Hertegard, S. & Gauffin, J. (1995) Glottal area and vibratory Patterns studied with simultaneous stroboscopy, flow glottography and electroglottography. J. Speech. Hear. Res. 38: 85–100

Hertel, N.T., Scheike, T., Juul, A., Main, K., Holm, K., Bach-Mortensen, N., Skakkebaek, N.E. & Muller, J.R. (1995) Kropsproportioner hos danske børn. Ugeskr. Laeger. 157: 6876–6881

Herzel, H., Berry, D., Titze, I.R. & Saleh, M. (1994) Analysis of vocal disorders with methods from nonlinear dynamics. J. Speech. Hear. Res. 37: 1008–1019

Hirano, M. (1989) Objective evaluation of the human voice: clinical aspects. Folia Phoniatr. 41: 89–144

Hirano, M., Kurita, S. & Nakashima, T. (1983) Growth, Development and Aging of Human Vocal Folds. In: Bless, D.M. & Abbs, J.H. (eds) Vocal Fold Physiology, College Hill Press, San Diego, California: 22–43

Hirano, M., Kiyokawa, K. & Kurita, S. (1988) Laryngeal Muscles and Glottic Shaping. In: Fujimura, O. ed. Vocal Physiology: Voice Production, Mezhanisms and Functions. Vol. 2. Raven Press, N.Y., pp 49–65

Hirose, H., Kiritani, H. & Imagawa, H. (1988) High-Speed Digital Image Analysis of Laryngeal Behavior in Running Speech. In: Vocal Physiology: Voice Production, Mechanisms and Functions. Vol. 2. Fujimura, O. (ed.) Raven Press, N.Y., pp 335–345

Hollien, H. (1983) In Search of Vocal Frequency Control Mechanisms. In: Bless, D.M. & Abbs, J.H. (eds) Vocal Fold Physiology. College-Hill Press, San Diego, California, pp 361–367

Hollien, H. & Malcik, E. (1967) Evaluation of cross-sectional studies of adolescent voice change in males. Speech Monogr. 34: 80–84

Hollien, H. & Shipp, T. (1972) Speaking fundamental frequency and chronologic age in males. J. Speech. Hear. Res. 15: 155–159

Hollien, H., Green, R. & Massey, K. (1994) Longitudinal research an adolescent voice change in males. J. Acoust. Soc. Am. 96: 2646–2654

International Phonetic Assoziation (1964) reprint from 1949: The Principles of the International Phonetic Assoziation. ed. Dept. Phonetics, Univ. College, London, W.C. 1

Kahane, J.C. (1982) Growth of the human prepubertal and pubertal larynx. J. Speech. Hear. Res 25: 446–455

Karlberg, P. & Taranger, J. (1976) The somatic development of children in a Swedish urban community. Acta Paediatr. Scand. Suppl. 256: 1–148

Karnell, M.P. (1989) Synchronized video stroboscopy and electroglottography. J. Voice 3: 68–75

Karnell, M.P. (1991) Laryngeal pertubationanalysis: minimum length of analysis window. J. Speech. Hear. Res. 34: 544–548

Kay Elemetrics Corp. (1993) Voice range profile model 4326. Operation manual. Pine Brook NJ

Kersing, W. (1983) De Stimmband Musculatur. Een Histologischeen histochemische Studie. Thesis. Utrecht. The Netherlands

Kitzing, P. (1979) Glottographisk Frekvensindikering. Thesis. University of Lund. Sweden

Kitzing, P. (1990) Clinical application of electroglottography. J. Voice 4: 238–249

Klingholz, F. & Martin, F. (1983) Die quantitative Auswertung der Stimmfeld-Messung. Sprache, Stimme, Gehör 7: 106–110

Klingholz, F., Jolk, A. & Martin, F. (1989) Stimmfeld-untersuchungen bei Knabenstimmen (Tölzer Knabenchor). Sprache, Stimme, Gehör 13: 107–111

Komyama, S., Watanabe, H. & Ryu, S. (1984) Phonetographic relationship between pitch and intensity of the human voice. Folia Phoniatr. 36: 1–7

Konzelmann, U., Moser, M. & Kittel, G. (1989) Stimmfeldmessungen bei Chorsängern vor und nach Stimmbelastung unter besonderer Berücksichtigung des Sängerformanten. Sprache, Stimme, Gehör 13: 112–118

Krabbe, S. (1989) Calcium homeostasis and mineralization in puberty. Dan. Med. Bull. 36: 113–124

Krusnevskaja, I.I. & Pedersen, M. (1992) Phonetograms of radiated voices in Chernobyl. Proc. XXI congr. Int. Ass. Logoped. Phoniatr. Hannover 16: 1–9

Kurita, S., Hirano, M., Mihashi, S. & Nakashima,' T. (1980) Layer structure of the vocal fold, age-dependant variation. Proc. XVIIIth congr. Int. Ass. Logoped. Phoniatr.: 537 539

Large, J. & Iwata, S. (1972) The male operatic head registers versus falsetto. Folia Phoniatr. 24: 19–29

Lecluse, F.L.E. (1977) Electroglottographie. Thesis. Utrecht. The Netherlands.

Loebell, E. (1968) Uber den klinishen Wert der Electroglottographie. Arch. Klin. Exp. Ohren Nasen Kehlkopfheilkd. 191: 760–764

Lundy, D.S., Roy, S., Casiano, R.R., Xue, J.W., Evans, J. (2000) Acoustic analysis of the singing and speaking voice in singing students. J Voice. 14(4): 490–493

Lykkesfeldt, G., Bennett, P., Lykkesfeldt, A.E., Micic, S., Moller, S. & Svenstrup, B. (1985) Abnormal androgen and oestrogen metabolism in men with steroid sulphatase defficiency and recessive x-linked ichthyosis. Clin. Endocrinol. 23: 385–3393

Marin, M.L., Tobias, M.L. & Kelley, D.B. (1990) Hormone-sensitive stages in the sexual differentiation of laryngeal muscle fiber in Xenopus laevis. Development 110: 703–711

McAllister, A., Sederholm, E., Sundberg, J. & Gramming, P. (1994) Relations between voice range profiles and physiological and perceptual voice characteristics in ten-year old children. J. Voice 8: 230–239

McGlone, R.E. & McGlone, J. (1972) Speaking fundamental frequency of eight-year-old girls. Folia Phoniatr. 24: 313–317

Meuser, W. & Nieschlag, W. (1977) Sex hormones and vocal register in adult men. Acta Endocrinol. Suppl. (Copenh.) 208: 61

Michel, J.F., Hollien, H. & Moore, P. (1966) Speaking fundamental frequency characteristics of 15, 16 and 17-year old girls. Lang. Speech 9: 46–51

Miranda, R., Sohrabji, F., Singh, M. & Toran-Allerand, D. (1996) Nerve growth factor (NGF) regulation of estrogen receptors in explant cultures of the developing forebrain. J. Neurobiol. 31: 77–87

Nastiuk, K.L. & Clayton, D.F. (1995) The canary androgen receptor mRNA is localized in the song control nuclei of the brain and is rapidly regulated by testosterone. J. Neurobiol. 26: 213–224

Niedzielska, G., Toman, D., Wroczek-Glijer, E. (1999) Hormonal conditioning of vocal changes in male. Otolaryngol Pol. 1999;53(4): 485–487

Pabon, J.P.H. (1991) Objective acoustic voice-quality parameters in the Computer phonetogram. J. Voice 5: 203–216

Pahn, J. & Pahn, E. (1991) Formblatt, Eigenschaften, Ablauf und Bedeutung des Tests der Sensibilitat formaler sprachlicher Elemente im Hinblick auf Perzeption und Produktion. Sprache, Stimme, Gehör 15: 19–23

Pedersen, M. (1974) A clinical examination of patients with benign tumors of the larynx, before and after microlaryngoscopy. Proc. XVIth congr. Int. Ass. Logopedics and Phoniatr.: 378–383

Pedersen, M. (1978) Electroglottography compared with synchronized stroboscopy in students of music. The study of sound, Tokyo 18: 423–434

Pedersen, M. (1991a) Computed phonetograms in adult patients with benign voice disorders before and after treatment with a non – sedating antihistamine (Loratadine). Folia Phoniatr. 43: 60–67

Pedersen, M. (1991b) Pilotstudie der Stimmfunktion vor und nach Behandlung von Hirngeschädigten. In: Gundermann, H. (ed.) Die Krankheit der Stimme, die Stimme der Krankheit. Fischer Verlag, Stuttgart: 162–171

Pedersen, M. (1991c) Die biologische Entwicklung der Stimme in der Pubertat. Bundesverband Deutscher Gesangpädagogen. Dokumentation ed. Detmold Hochschule für Musik: 28–37

Pedersen, M. (1992) Bookreview. C.E. Seashore. Psychology of Music. Folia Phoniatrica 44: 312

Pedersen, M. V (1993) A longitudinal pilot study an phonetograms/voice profiles in pre-pubertal choir boys. Clin. Otolaryngol. 18: 488–491

Pedersen, M. (1995) Stimmfunktion vor und nach Behandlung von Hirngeschä-digten, mit Stroboskopie, Phonetographie und Luftstrom–Analyse durchgeführt. Sprache, Stimme, Gehör 19: 84–89

Pedersen, M. I (1977) Electroglottography compared with synchronized stroboscopy in normal persons. Folia Phoniatr. 29: 191–199

Pedersen, M. & Lindskov Hansen, H. (1986) Computerized phonetograms for
clinical use. Folia phoniatr. Proc. XXth Congr. of IALP, Tokyo: 170–171

Pedersen, M. & Moller, S. (1987) A transport globulin, serum hormon binding
globulin, as a predicting factor of voice change in puberty? Proc. Xl Int.
Congr. Phonetic Sciences, Tallinn 4: 296–299

Pedersen, M. & Munk, E. (1983) Register examination during mutation in the
Copenhagen Boys Choir.Proc. XIX congr. Int. Ass. Logopedics and Phoniatr.: 686–687

Pedersen, M., Eriksen, K. & Heramb, S. (1980) A follow up study of patients
with voice disorders. Proc. XVIII congr. Int. Ass. Logopedics and Phoniatr.
Washington 1: 621–626

Pedersen, M., Kitzing, P., Krabbe, S. & Heramb, S. (1982) The change of voice
during puberty in 11 to 16 year old choir singers measured with electroglottographic fundamental frequency analysis and compared to other phenomena of puberty. Acta Otolaryngol. Suppl. (Stockh.) 385: 189–192

Pedersen, M., Lindskov Hansen, T., Lindskov Hansen, H. & Munk, E. (1984) A
Phonetograph for Use in Clinical Praxis. Acta Otolaryngol. Suppl. (Stockh.)
412: 138

Pedersen, M. IV, Møller, S., Krabbe, S., Munk, E. & Bennett, P. (1985a) A multivariate statistical analysis of voice phenomena related to puberty in choir
boys. Folia Phoniatr. 37: 271–278

Pedersen, M., Moller, S., Eriksen, K. & Sondergaard, U. (1985b) Quantitative
and qualitative diagnoses of children with voice disorders. New Dimen.
Otorhinolaryngol. Head Neck Surg 2: 470–471

Pedersen, M. III, Møller, S., Krabbe, S. & Bennett, P. (1986a) Fundamental
voice frequency measured by electroglottography during continuous speech.
A new exact secondary sex characteristic in boys in puberty. Int. J. Pediatr.
otorhinolaryngol. 11: 21–27

Pedersen, M., Moller, S., Krabbe, S., Bennett, P. & Munk, E. (1986b) Phonetograms in Choir Boys Compared with Voice Categories, Somatic Puberty and
Androgen Development. J. Res Sing 9: 39–49

Pedersen, M., Hacki, T. & Loebell, E. (1988a) Videostroboscopy of choir boys
in puberty. Video presentation. Medizinische Hochschule. Hannover

Pedersen, M., Seidner, W. & Wendler, J. (1988b) Collection and processing of
voice field data. Methodical approaches. Proc. XV congr. Union of European Phoniatricians. Erlangen: 107

Pedersen, M. II, Møller, S., Krabbe, S., Bennett, P. & Svenstrup, B. (1990a) Fundamental voice frequency in female puberty measured with electroglottography during continuous speech as a secondary sex characteristic. A comparison between voice, pubertal stages, oestrogens and androgens. Int. J. Pediatr. Otorhinolaryngol. 20: 17–24

Pedersen, M., Moller, S. & Bennett, P. (1990b) Voice Categories Compared with Phonetograms, Androgens, Estrogens and Puberty Stages in 8–19 Year Old Girls. J. Research Singing 13: 1–4

Rihkanen, H., Leinonen, L., Hiltunen, T. & Kangas, J. (1994) Spectral pattern recognition of improved voice quality. J. Voice 8: 320–326

Rodriguez-Sierra, J. (1986) Extended organizational effects of estrogen at puberty. Ann. N. Y. Acad. Sci. 474: 293–306

Roed, J., Larsen, R.B. & Ibsen, K.K. (1989) The heights of a population of children in greater Copenhagen aged 7–18 years in 1981 and 1985. Ugeskrift Laeger 159: 895–897

Rothenberg, M. (1992) A multichannel electroglottograph. J. Voice 6: 36–43

Roubeau, B., Chevrie-Muller, C. & Arabia-Guidet, C. (1987) Electroglottographic study of the change of voice registers. Folia Phoniatr. 39: 280–289

Russell, A., Penny, L. & Pemberton, C. (1995) Speaking fundamental frequency changes over time in women: a longitudinal study. J. Speech. Hear. Res. 38: 101–109

Sataloff, R.T. (1995) Genetics of the voice. J. Voice 9: 20–26

Sato, K. & Hirano, M. (1995) Histologic investigations of the macula flava of the human vocal fold. Ann. Otol. Rhinol. Laryngol. 104: 138–143

Schönhärl, E. (1960) Die Stroboskopie in der praktischen Laryngologie. Thieme. Stuttgart

Schulz-Coulon, H.J. & Klingholz, F. (1988) Objective und semiobjective Untersuchungen der Stimme. In: Proc. XV Congr. Union of European Phoniatricians Erlangen: 3–88

Schutte, H.K. (1995) Phonetogram: voice capacities and clinical value. Abstracts, Ist. World Conf. of Voice, Oporto, Portugal: 265

Schutte, H.K. & Seidner, W. (1983) Recommendation by the Union of European Phoniatricians (UEP): Standardizing voice area measurement/phonetography. Folia Phoniatr. 35: 286–288

Seashore, C.E. (1938) Psychology of music. McGraw-Hill, NY, USA. (Republication Dover 1967)

Seidner, W. & Schutte, H.K. (1981) Standardisierungsvorschlag Stimmfeld Messung/Phonetographie. Proc. IX Congr. Union of European Phoniatricians. Amsterdam: 88–94

Seidner, W. & Wendler, J. (1982) Die Sängerstimme. Wilhelmshafen, Heinrichshofen: 174–178

Seidner, W., Kruger, H. & Wernecke, K.D. (1985). Numerische Auswertung spektraler Stimmfelder. Sprache, Stimme, Gehör 9: 10–13

Siegel, W. ed. (1994) Proceedings, Int. Computer Music Conference, Århus. Denmark.

Smith, S. (1954) Remarks on the physiology of the vocal cords. Folia Phoniatr. 6: 166–179

Smith, S. (1981) Research on the principle of electroglottography. Folia phoniatr. 33: 1–10

Strel'Chyonok, O.A. & Vihko, R. (1985) Specific steroid-binding glycoproteins of human bloodplasma. Novel data an their structure and function. J. Steroid. Biochem. 35: 519–534

Stürzeberger, E., Wagner, H., Becker, R., Rauhut, A. & Seidner, W. (1982) Einrichtung zur simultanen Registrierung von Stimmfeld und hohem Sängerformant. HNO-Praxis Leipzig; 7: 223–226

Sulter, A.M., Schutte, H.M. & Miller, D.G. (1995) Differences in Phonetogram Features Between Male and Female Subjects With and Without Vocal Training. J. Voice 9: 363–377

Sundberg, J. (1987) The science of the singing voice. Northern Illinois Univ. Press. Sundberg, J. (1994) Perceptual aspects of singing. J. Voice 8: 106–122

Svec, J. & Pesak, J. (1994) Vocal breaks from modal to falsetto register. Folia Phoniatr. 46: 97–103

Tanner, J.M. & Whitehouse, R.H. (1976) Clinical longitudinal standards for height, weight, height velocity and stages of puberty. Arch. Dis. Child. 51: 170–179

Titze, I.R. (1994) Toward standards in acoustic analysis of voice. J. Voice 8: 1–7

Tobias, M.L. & Kelley, D.B. (1995) Sexual differentiation and hormonal regulation of the laryngeal synapse in Xenopus laevis. J. Neurobiol. 28: 515–526

Tobias, M.L., Marin, M.L. & Kelley, D.B. (1991) Temporal constraints, androgen directed laryngeal masculinization in Xenopus laevis. Dev. Biol. 147: 260–270

Truuverk, C. & Pedersen, M. (1992) A pilot study of phonetograms compared with menopausal estrogens and androgens in 4 sopranoes in World Festival Choir. Abstracts XXInd Congr. Int. Ass. Logopedics Phoniatr. Folia Phoniatr. 1–2: 85

Van Lierde, K.M., Claeys, S., De Bodt, M., Van Cauwenberge, P. (2006) Responses of the female vocal quality and resonance in professional voice users taking oral contraceptive pills: a multiparameter approach. Laryngoscope 116 (10): 1894–1898

Vilkman, E., Sonninen, A. & Hurme, P. (1986) Observations on voice productions by means of Computer voice profiles. Proc. XX congr. Int. Ass. Logopedics and Phoniatr, Tokyo: 370–371

Vilkman, E., AIku, P. & Laukkanen, A.-M. (1995) Vocal-fold collision as a differentiator between registers in the low-pitch range. J. Voice 9: 66–73

Vuorenkoski, V., Lenko, H.L., Tjernlund, P., Vuorenkoski, L. & Perheentupe, J. (1978) Fundamental frequency during normal and abnormal growth, and after androgen treatment. Arch. Dis. Child. 53: 201–209

Walker, J.M., Williams, D.M., Harries, M., Hacking, J. & Hughes, I.A. (1993) A study of the mechanisms of normal voice maturation in pubertal boys. Pediatr. Res. 33(suppl 5): S 84

Weiss, D.A. (1950) The pubertal change of the human voice.Folia Phoniatr. 2: 126–159

Wendler, J. (1989) Basic equipment for voice diagnosis. Newsletter. Int. Fed. Otorhinolaryngol. Socictics. Fcb.-March: 3

Wendler, J. & Seidner, W. (1987) Entwicklung der Stimme. In: Lehrbuch der Phoniatrie. Thieme Verlag: 164–169

Wendler, J., Koppen, K. & Fischer, S. (1988) The validity of stroboscopic data in terms of quantitative measuring. Folia Phoniatr. 40: 297–302

Wiskirska-Wonica, B., Obrebowski, A., Wojciechowska, A., Walczak, M. (2006) The local and sensual conditions of delay of voice breaking in adolescent boys. Otolaryngol Pol. 60(3): 397–400

Young, M.C., Robinson, J.A., Read, G.F., Riad-Fahmy, D. & Hughes, I.A. (1988) 170 H-progesterone rythms in congenital adrenal hypoplasia. Arch. Dis. Child 63: 617–623

Yukizane, S., Yamakawa, R., Murakami, T., Kato, H. & Niikawa, N. (1994) A 15-year-old girl with pubertal masculinization due to bilateral gonadoblastoma and 45, X/46, X, +Mar Karyotype. Kurume Med. J. 41: 155–159

Original Communications

The permission of the following copyright owners to reproduce original articles is gratefully acknowledged:

- Karger (Folia Phoniatrica, Reports of IALP Conferences)
- Elsevier (Int. J. Pediatric Otorhinolaryngology)
- Blackwell (Clinical Otolaryngology)

Abbreviations

DHEAS	Dihydroepiandrosterone sulphate
EGG	Electroglottography
El	Oestrone
E2	Oestradiol
E1SO4	Oestrone sulphate
F0	F0 mean fundamental frequency in running speech in a reading situation of a standard text
F0	F0-range frequency variation in semitones in running speech in a reading situation of a standard text (=voice range)
LTAS	Long-term averaged spectrogram
Octaves:	German description: C-c-cl-c2-c3, American: C3 = c, C4 = cl, C5 = c2 etc.

SHBG	Sex hormone binding globulin
ST	Semitone in the octave (as on a piano, 12 per octave), defined from the phonetogram
SPL	Sound pressure level
Total pitch range	The range from the lowest to the highest semitone in the phonetogram

Index